Kavery Nambisan was born in Kodagu district, Karnataka. She did her medical studies at St John's Medical College, Bangalore and her higher surgical studies in the UK. After obtaining the Fellowship of the Royal College of Surgeons (FRCS) from London, she worked predominantly in the rural parts of Uttar Pradesh, Bihar, Tamil Nadu and Karnataka. She has also worked as a governing council member of the Association of Rural Surgeons of India.

She has written seven novels, including *The Scent of Pepper*, *The Story That Must Not Be Told* and *A Town Like Ours*. She has also written several books for children. This is her first long non-fiction work.

Kavery was married to the poet and writer Vijay Nambisan. She lives and works in Kodagu district and can be reached at kavery.nambisan@gmail.com

A LUXURY CALLED HEALTH

A DOCTOR'S JOURNEY THROUGH THE ART, THE SCIENCE AND THE TRICKERY OF MEDICINE

Kavery Nambisan

SPEAKING
TIGER

SPEAKING TIGER BOOKS LLP
125A, Ground Floor, Shahpur Jat, near Asiad Village,
New Delhi 110049

Published by Speaking Tiger Books in paperback 2021

ISBN: 978-93-5447-069-1
eISBN: 978-93-5447-070-7

10 9 8 7 6 5 4 3 2 1

Typeset in Adobe Garamond Pro by SÜRYA, New Delhi
Printed at Shree Maitrey Printech Pvt. Ltd., Noida

Doctors and Patients:
For you
Because of you

'Fortunately, when religion was strong and science weak, men mistook magic for medicine; now, when science is strong and religion weak, men mistake medicine for magic.'—Thomas Szasz; *The Second Sin*

Contents

	Introduction	1
	Prologue	12
1.	Learning	18
2.	'Go West'	30
3.	Internship	41
4.	Truly Rural	49
5.	Bones	56
6.	England	61
7.	Chirugia	67
8.	Safaai Karmachari	73
9.	Ancestor Worship	78
10.	Plumbing Away…	89
11.	The National Health Service	96
12.	Why Not Bihar?	100
13.	Speaking of Krishna…	112
14.	City Lights	130
15.	Change Is Inevitable	138

16. A Hol(e)y Health Care 145
17. The Rural Hospital 150
18. Corporate Medical Wisdom 162
19. Home Building 172
20. Rural Wounds, Urban Ulcers 178
21. Doctoring Reality 188
22. My Clinic 205
23. The Four Prongs of Illness 212
24. The Food We Eat 216
25. The Environment 227
26. Can Your Job Kill You? 232
27. The SFL Triangle 237
28. Mothers, Daughters, Wives 246
29. From 11 November 2016… 256
30. …to 9 August 2017 276
31. A Virus Strikes 284
32. A World View 294
Afterword 304
Acknowledgements 305

Introduction

As I prepare to let go of this book, I realize with dismay that I have spent a major portion of two decades convincing myself of its needlessness. I like medical work, and I like writing fiction. But I find it hard to summon the enthusiasm required to put down large chunks of my life into words that others might read. It does not permit me to imagine stories and create characters—which I love doing. There is also the fear of what self-examination might yield.

By way of introduction, here is an unsettling scene from Dostoevsky's *The Brothers Karamazov,* a novel I read every few years. There is one scene in the novel where a boy, Ilyusha, lies terminally ill in bed in his impoverished home. The father is trying desperately to save him, his physically disabled sister and their mother who is a melancholic neurotic. Through the noble efforts of a rich woman, a reputed physician has arrived to see Ilyusha.

The doctor enters their home, making obvious his distaste and scorn for the job at hand; he does a cursory examination of the boy and walks out. At the doorway stands the father: questioning, pleading with his eyes for a miracle that will save his son. The doctor is irritated by the poor, cringing man. With elaborate sarcasm he proclaims that since it is a very serious condition, it would be best to take the boy to Syracuse, in Sicily, for convalescence. He adds that the physically disabled daughter should be taken to some place in the Caucasus and his wife to a famed psychiatrist in Paris. He knows full well that it is beyond their means and yet he cruelly recommends it. His advice can only make Ilyusha's father feel that he is not doing enough.

Kolya, Ilyusha's friend, is waiting outside, as anxious as the family. He has heard the physician, sized up the situation and is furious. Here is how the scene plays out when the father hears the doctor's suggestion:

'Doctor! Doctor! Don't you see?' he exclaims, pointing to the bare log walls of the house.

'Ah, that is not my business,' the doctor grins. 'I have only said what science can say to your questions. As for the rest… to my regret…' He looks uneasily at the dog Perzivon which is waiting at the doorway with Kolya.

'Don't worry, Leech, my dog won't bite you!' cuts in Kolya, abruptly. (Later, Kolya declares he used the word 'leech' instead of 'doctor' purposely, and 'meant it as an insult'.)

The doctor, flabbergasted, is unable to give a fitting reply. Kolya continues to address him as Leech. Shamed and irate, the doctor climbs into his ostentatious carriage and slinks away.

I have merely given a window-peep's description of the fictional scene so powerfully described a century and a half ago. It is perhaps not the image of the quintessential doctor. But it provokes reflection upon a craft which entitles qualified doctors to attempt the cure, or at least the amelioration of the misery caused by sickness. Our profession itself merits self-examination and I have taken on the uneasy task of attempting to portray it. What follows is coloured by my own experience, backed by observation and collected detail. For the positives and the negatives of the telling, I take the credit and the blame.

*

My training has been solely in Western medicine, or Allopathy. It is based on the meticulous study of the human body, its chemical composition, the physics, the geometry of alignment and the organization of organs into systems which function in accord with each other. This is followed by the study of the *why* and *how* of every disease, and the ways in which we can set it right.

Claude Bernard, the 19th-century French physiologist, wrote a treatise describing the 'milieu interior' or the inner harmony of the body and its ability to adjust to a changing external environment. The lungs receive oxygen from the atmosphere and deliver it to the heart; the heart pumps oxygen-rich blood to every organ; the digestive system breaks food into simple molecules which dissolve into the blood stream to provide energy; the brain sends messages through its neural network, signalling us to act in different ways.

The body is a finely tuned instrument which must also make constant, delicate alterations to suit the rhythm of the outside world: the skin adjusts to external heat and cold by controlling the blood flowing to it, ensuring that it can cool off or warm up quickly. This is similar to a thermostat which controls the temperature in a room or building. The ability to maintain this balance, within and without, is the milieu interior of Claude Bernard. In other words, homeostasis, that is common to all forms of life. The American physiologist W.B. Cannon described it as 'the wisdom of the body'. If homeostasis is maintained, there is life. If it is disrupted, there is disease, perhaps death. We see this mechanism in all of nature—in every atom, cell, molecule, organ, organism—in technology, and in communities. The computer is a standard example of several components operating in synchrony. As I type, it follows commands, and self-regulates within its metal framework while also reacting to my constantly changing finger-typed commands, or to an external disc or drive inserted into it for new functions like the playing of music or film.

Nature provides a seemingly perfect balance: the migration

of birds, the hibernation of animals, the warming and cooling of different regions, the level of water in an open well are examples of homeostasis. Irregularities happen, resulting in periodic cataclysms: floods, drought, cyclones, forest fires, wars; or in the body, disease. This disruption is set right through the required adjustments which revive the dynamic equilibrium so essential to life. The inter-connectedness between Nature and all forms of life is mutually beneficial.

The human body, which can also be looked at as a part of Nature, is a marvel of creation. So are societies—groups of people forming a community, a country, a republic like India, which is a *created* marvel of variety. Through the years it has suffered several episodes of ill-health and nervous breakdown. Some were serious, tragic, indelible disasters which left us scarred, but our republic succeeded in bouncing back to health every time. When the harmony of coexistence and mutual respect between people is eroded, society crumbles; when we cease to respect nature, misuse and abuse its bounty, the weather patterns change, resulting in natural catastrophes; when we abuse the equilibrium of the body, there is ill health and disease. All these factors might eventually decide the fate of the human race, and even that of every other form of life. Nature is not always perfect—at times it is playfully imperfect—but the only demand that it makes on us is that we respect and retain the connections. Health, like security and peace, lies in maintaining harmony within and without. When health has been disturbed, doctors step in. It is their job to restore it.

The Westernized or allopathic medicine which we widely follow is relatively new in our part of the world. For millennia, non-European societies thrived and progressed without the influence of Western thought. Most of Asia used traditional systems of healing which were more in tune with nature: Ayurveda, Siddha, Unani, Yoga and Naturopathy; Chinese, Tibetan and Japanese medicines were for long preferred in

Asian countries. Homoeopathy, which originated in Europe, became popular in many parts of Asia in the 19th century.

Ayurveda ('Life Knowledge') is the ancient system most prevalent in southern parts of India, particularly Kerala. The oldest known texts, dating back from the 6th to the 2nd century BCE, are *Susrutha Samhita*, *Charaka Samhita* and Nagarjuna's *Madhyamaka* or the Middle Path. The body is believed to be made of the five elements and three doshas (vata, pitta and kapha). An equilibrium between the doshas and a balance of the elements are considered essential for well-being. Illness is diagnosed by observing the pulse, urine, stool, tongue, speech, appearance, gait, vision, mouth and body odour. Thus, observation is the mainstay of diagnosis. Colleges, hospitals and clinics of Ayurveda are popular in Kerala, and are gaining popularity in the rest of the country, too, although, increasingly, in ways that may damage rather than maintain or restore the health of individuals, society and the country.

Homoeopathy is dismissed by many as an ineffective pseudo-science, and at best a placebo. My own experience has been different: years ago, our daughter's recurrent throat infections, which did not respond to cough mixtures and antibiotics, led us to a homoeopath. At eight-thirty in the morning there were twenty or more patients waiting their turn to be seen by this bespectacled monk. He sat behind a wooden table stacked with jars and bottles, handing out individually wrapped sachets of sweet powders. His palatable and inexpensive treatment cured my daughter. I have used Homoeopathy myself and often suggest it for children who suffer frequent throat infections.

Samuel Hahnemann of Germany was the first proponent of Homoeopathy. He was a physician trained in Western medicine towards the end of the 18th century. Seeing the toxic effects of allopathic medicines of his time, he was frustrated enough to give up his practice and later formulated the theory that 'Like cures like'. A substance which causes symptoms of a disease in healthy persons could cure the same symptoms in the sick, if used in minute doses. Homoeopathy came to India when eight Jesuit priests from Europe arrived in the coastal town of Mangalore, Karnataka, to teach French and mathematics at the newly established St Aloysius College. One of them was Father Muller who was experienced in the use of homoeopathic medicines. When students fell ill, he treated them with his little pills. Every evening he sat beneath a banyan tree near the college and saw patients. One day he was asked to treat a woman with leprosy. Soon many people, particularly the poor, came to him for help and so he started a dispensary. Father Muller's Hospital which combined the use of Homoeopathy and Allopathy was established in 1883 and still exists. Remarkably, it has retained a certain nobility of spirit so rare now in medical institutions. Homoeopathy is a particular favourite of Bengalis. You are sure to find a homoeopath in any locality of a city that has more than a dozen Bengali families. Chittaranjan Park in Delhi ('Little Bengal', more or less) has two well-known homoeopaths. The queues outside their homes can make any doctor envious.

Unani (Yunan in Arabic) had its origins in West Asia in the 11th century. It combines the wisdom of many physicians, including the famed Al Razi, Al Zahrawi and Ibn Nafis. It is based on the concept of four humours, roughly corresponding to the phlegm, blood, yellow bile and black bile of ancient Greece. It was brought to India in the 13th century by the Delhi Sultanate and became popular under the patronage of the Mughal kings. Unani physicians (hakims) held eminent positions in the royal courts for several centuries. The Azizis of Lucknow and the Sharifis of Delhi were two prominent families which incorporated the wisdom of Ayurveda and Allopathy with Unani medicine. In all our metros and in many small towns, you will still find centres of Unani.

Siddha medicine evolved from Dravidian traditions in Tamil Nadu. It aims for perfect health by following a physical, mental and social code of ethics. The original masters were believed to have supernatural or Siddhic powers gained by the practice of meditation, yoga and spiritual living. They use herbs and sometimes powdered animal bones and minerals or massage and pressure methods or thokkam* in the treatment of injury and disease. Over four thousand diseases, including those linked to genetic factors, are listed among those that can be cured by the Siddhars, without causing undesired side-effects.

Medical tourism is relatively new in our corporate hospitals but it has quietly flourished in the field of alternate medicine, particularly with Ayurveda and yoga. Some of our tenaciously fit yogis found instant favour among the Westerners. The combination of stretching exercises through yoga, controlled breathing and massage worked wonders on the Westerner reared on an obscenely rich diet of meats, butter and lard-rich desserts and sugary drinks. I first heard about the yoga gurus in England in the mid-1980s and once attended a bizarre 'group-healing' session in London. It was held in a darkly curtained drawing room of a home. The saffron-clad European guru was seated on an ornate chair with velvet draperies. He was explaining the joys of transcendental meditation to an earnest bunch of women and a few men, trying to impress them with words like 'aura', 'levitation', and urging them to recognize the 'kundalini' and develop the 'Om personality'. I was not inclined towards a transcendental experience of any sort and this European fake strengthened my disbelief. At least, since I had gone as the guest of a friend, I did not shell out any money.

---

*Thokkam is a popular method of giving pain relief in musculo-skeletal problems of all kinds and has been practised for thousands of years. It is the application of pressure on specific 'energy storage' points in the body, of which there are twelve. It is a difficult skill which requires the identification of the exact spot for the application of pressure. The smallest error can lead to aggravation of the problem.

Publicity stunts in yoga are the rage now but we do not need to enact en masse in playgrounds and maidans to show off to the rest of humanity. It dilutes the essence of a great way of life that belonged to our ancestors. Notwithstanding the charlatans in their many guises, the popularity of yoga is largely due to teachers such as B.K.S. Iyengar, Sri Krishnamacharya, the teachers of the Munger school of yoga, as also a few more recent, populist gurus like Baba Ramdev, Sri Sri Ravi Shankar and the rest. Unfortunately, this latter variety of businessmen-gurus have mixed it not only with big money and the cult of personality but also religious prejudice and exclusionary politics—everything contrary to health and harmony.

As Allopathy loses its charm due to a variety of reasons, there has been a revival of the ancient methods of healing. But profiteering has infected the medical bloodstream and alternate medical practitioners are catching up. Some Ayurvedic centres in India are also run (almost) exclusively for foreigners. I recently went to a place that is a hotspot for Russians. My reason for going was partly curiosity but also an expectation of reviving a yoga routine I have followed for years. The young therapists and masseurs, the doctors and other staff are given lessons in Russian; the reading room is stocked exclusively with Russian novels and magazines. The owner of the establishment is frank about discouraging locals who, he says, are more skeptical about the benefits of treatment. I was accepted perhaps as a professional colleague, or more likely, because it was off-season for the Russians. The treatment itself, a combination of saathvic food, exercise and breathing technique, was useful.

The shift from traditional medical systems to Allopathy happened gradually between the 18th and 20th century. The scientific spirit of enquiry, learning and verification scored over ancient knowledge systems which lacked the concept of research and documentation. The making of medicinal drugs using chemical compounds and minerals started in Europe.

With the ability to transport them, these tablets, syrups and injections could be sent to different parts of the world. Pharmaceutical industries began to prosper. But right until the mid-19th century, the serious side-effects of these drugs used to frighten patients away. The medicines used to treat serious ailments were either too toxic, or ineffective unless served up in large doses. And the end result of many a serious illness—plague, smallpox, tuberculosis, syphilis—was lethal.

Nonetheless, the pills and potions began to catch on. Doctors and pharmacists started concocting 'elixirs'. It would at least bring the hope back into a patient's eyes while the physician retained the secret of the mysterious-sounding ingredients in his medicines. He became adept at prescriptions written in Latin (and now, in India, in deliberately, breathtakingly illegible English—always English—that few mortals outside a chemist's shop can decipher). Alcohol, the great inducer of temporary well-being, began to be used as a vehicle in all liquid-based medicines. There was also opium and its derivative morphine, one of the few drugs of real value—but for the fact that opiates are addictive. Pharmacists compounded the medicines: so much of a powder by weight dissolved in sugary alcohol and flavoured with spices or the essence of fruit.

Western medicine came to India through apothecaries who came with the traders of the East India Company. Their merchants landed in India after a long, perilous voyage. Unaccustomed to the tropical climate, difficult terrain, endless journeys within the country and the strange food, they fell prey to diseases like malaria, kalaazar, cholera and tuberculosis. As the number of British in India increased and their families began to join them, more doctors were needed. So began the Indian Medical Service (IMS) in 1835 which offered a short course of medical training followed by examinations held in London. Their medical practice was referred to in India as 'doctory' (or 'dactri' in Hindi heartlands) and their work was initially restricted to the British in India; Indians continued to rely on vaidyars, hakims and other practitioners. As wars became more frequent, the treatment of injured and ailing native soldiers also became imperative. A Subordinate Medical Service (SMS) was set up in Calcutta and later in Madras and Bombay. Subsequently, a medical college was established in Calcutta and soon after in the other two Presidencies.

At first, only the Christians and Parsis showed any inclination for medical training since most Hindus were either averse to human dissection or they were unlettered. This changed when Pandit Madhusudan Gupta performed the first human dissection in 1836, and thus broke through the barrier to training in Western medicine. Native practitioners started to make use of the thermometer, stethoscope, the microscope and other Western aides to enhance their skills.

The vaidyars and hakims held interactions with the British doctors and worked side by side with them. The lack of scientific proof and research in these Eastern systems subsequently led to their attrition and decline. By the mid-19th century, the British looked upon all systems other than Allopathy as quackery and stopped supporting them in any way. The royal families and several wealthy Indians began to seek allopathic care. As more medical colleges came up, the trust in indigenous forms of medicine began to fade.

At Independence, we had twenty-two medical colleges in India. Western concepts of science and thought flowed freely to the east but Western medicine did not reach a vast majority of our people who resided outside of the cities. They still don't. In almost every major hospital in a big city it is a common sight to see groups of bewildered villagers and small-town folk. They struggle to cope with the ostentation, the complexities of modern hospitals, and the formidable challenge of shelling out exorbitant fees to avail treatment. Families of patients with serious illnesses sleep outside the hospital gates, on pavements or in hastily constructed shacks to while away anxious weeks or months—cooking, washing, sleeping in the open, waiting to go back to their homes and to work. The so-called 'charitable beds' provided by many private hospitals are but an eye-wash. Seventy-five years of great medical and economic advances have made no difference to these multitudes.

Over the decades, before Independence and beyond it, we chose to look away from age-old therapies, embraced Western medicine and progressed with great speed to where we are now. The human body is imbued with its own wisdom. Like so much of Nature, it forgives. But how well do we handle this body, this miracle of creation, this locomotive thinking machine that is so well articulated that it can move with fluid grace? And what is it that brings on disease to knock it off balance, and make us run to medical practitioners for help? I began my own medical career in earnest, full of hope and excitement about the limitless possibilities which lay before me. I was quite unaware of the realities of the medical world. That I discovered bit by bit.

I wonder why I ventured into writing this book. Writing, like all of art, is 'performance' on display and ultimately, risky business. Doctoring, which is the subject of this book, is also risky. The innumerable occasions in a doctor's career when she is confronted by a patient whose life trembles on the edge and she is the one who must reach out and rescue—the fluttering of the doctor's heart at such moments needs no mention. I am trying to open windows to some interesting moments of the doctoring business. I speak of what I know. I applaud and criticize so that we may understand better—a little better—what our real duties are. Allopathy is not the sole remedy for human suffering. Individual skills, commitment and courage are not enough. We need to remind society about the need to feel responsible for good health—for *everybody's* good health—and we need to remind our governments that healthy citizens are more important than a fat GDP.

Prologue

The letter was written on a light blue aerogramme costing five English pence. The three long paragraphs filled almost all of the writing space. Was I happy with it? Not quite, I think, for I told no one.

Away it went. I immersed myself in the routine tensions of the medical world in which I was something of a novice, not five years into the trade of cutting and sewing. One evening on returning to my room in Liverpool after work I saw a long cream-coloured envelope that had been slipped beneath my door, the way all my letters were delivered. Breaking open the red wax GOVERNMENT OF INDIA seal, I read.

> Dear Doctor,
>
> I am in receipt of your letter dated _____ and have noted its contents. India will prosper because of the many decisions I have taken and the programmes I have initiated. The majority of people are entirely happy with my leadership. A few ungrateful persons choose to leave this great country in order to escape to the west for material gains. However, India will earn its well-deserved place in the world and be an example for others to follow.
>
> It appears to me that you are trying to tell me how to run the country. I do not need advice from people like you.
>
> Signed
>
> The Prime Minister of India.

Mortified, I concealed the letter in the kitchen cupboard. I had been told to mind my own business. Having fretted for a few days, I took it out of its hiding place and tore it to shreds. It might have been panic, or the fear of revealing my foolishness to any other person. I have since learnt to carry my stupidities lightly on my shoulders and can even write about them. If I stop to think what made me send that letter, I might begin to understand many of the decisions which shaped my life. (I regret not having preserved that famous reply from Indira Gandhi. Perhaps the faded aerogramme on which I wrote the letter that earned the reply lives somewhere in the national archives.)

A year later, I was back in India and we were at lunch in our home. A friend of my father had come the previous day and the conversation veered towards politics, as it always did—my father and his friend being loyal to different political parties. Emergency was over but it was still a hot topic, and one of the few matters about which my father and his friend had similar views. On an impulse I told them about my letter. Exclamations of surprise and incredulity all round, and a smile on my father's face. He did not say a word. His friend, a man I admired very much, asked me, 'Is that why you came back?'

*

Three years earlier and a few months before I left for the UK to pursue my surgical training, a certain young man asked an astrologer about my future. After getting a few details of my horoscope from him, the astrologer predicted that my life would be most beautiful. He did not elaborate why and how it would be so. He gushed about it, but added that there was also terrible sadness in store for me. I think he was, in a way, warning the young man: *Avoid danger*. Young men in love never listen, of course.... But that is a different story, of no use to anyone but me and mine.

The fortune-teller wished to tell me more, in person, but the meeting never happened, which is just as well. I do not believe in weakly reasoned assumptions about some people being luckier than others; fortune is never partial, barring that which we come with when we are born. As a doctor I have seen many a life slip away into silence when it could have been pulled back, should have been pulled back. The prevalence of disease depends on many external factors, like too little or too much wealth, the availability or lack of medical care, and for some, the soul-destroying stresses of an unkind life. None of this is about good or bad fortune. It is about the kind of world we have ended up making.

*

My first brush with medicine, I've been told, was when I wasn't yet three. It was late afternoon and the children were at play in the wide open spaces outside the house. My mother noticed that I wasn't joining the fun, and found me hot and flushed with a raging fever. Tucking me into bed, she watched in horror my eyes go blank and my limbs flaccid. By the time my father could be beckoned from the paddy-threshing yard, the convulsions had set in. The nearest doctor was in town, 16 kilometres away. Warm blankets, cold water sprinkled over the face, prayers—nothing worked. The breathing became shallow, jerky and then stopped. With a loud moan my father lifted me in his arms. 'She's gone!'

Just then my grandfather, farmer, veterinary doctor and hard drinker, walked in through the gate swinging the customary bottle of toddy by a string around its neck. Having just visited the little shack—or club—where he enjoyed a few drinks with his friends, he was well-oiled within. Rushing to the cowshed where a corner had been portioned off as his dispensary, he grabbed a bottle of mustard-green liquid which he had recently brewed for his veterinary patients and poured a few drops into my mouth. I recovered in less than an hour.

My belief in astrologers is scant but I trust my grandfather's wisdom. A bit too much or too little of that bovine therapy made me what I am.

I was born in my mother's home, in one of the many bedrooms with a single small window through which my father peeped as the local midwife and my grandmother assisted my arrival into the world. Doctors were not sought for something as natural as childbirth. Kethi, the Yerava woman who assisted the delivery with my grandmother, was a household name. She was also a regular with us, her services required several times a year in that family of four parents and nineteen children. My birth was uneventful. Kethi was paid the usual fee of one rupee and an old sari. As an afterthought, my grandmother also gave her a plump hen from the chicken coop.

I have tried hard to think myself back to that moment when I fell off my mother but cannot, and instead fill it with scenes from my imagination. The beginning of my *ability* to remember is clear in memory. Not long after the attack of febrile fits, I became conscious of myself as a person. 'This is Me,' I said to my reflection in the mirror. 'This is who I am.' That three-year-old looks at me sometimes. I cannot hold her questioning gaze for too long. Instead, I take her on my lap. 'I'll do it. One day I'll do it,' I say to her, hugging her small shoulders, stroking her hair, feeling the smallness of bones in her hands and feet. 'One day I'll do it.'

I have had raging arguments, fights even, with various stages of my previous self; and I've had moments of quiet togetherness, when we have laughed at each other. It does not happen often. How can it, you cannot summon your past self with a snap of your fingers and say, 'Come here and answer for yourself.' Nowadays, with that three-year-old, I am silent. Her eyes are too clear and questioning.

*

Skimming thus over my past, I evade something important and which the fortune-teller would have said differently had he really known: that I would carry sadness like a heavy stone in my heart. It has weighted everything—at home, in hospitals, in life's gardens and in its wastelands. I first knew sadness when my mother told me all about being a big girl who must never do bad things because god only forgave bad things in babies and I was not a baby but a strapping five-year-old, perfectly capable of telling good from bad. I *wanted* to be good but could never be good all the time, and it saddened me. I said my 'sorry' to whoever it was up there in the clouds playing god and then went on to live my life the way I wanted to live it. More or less.

I had good parents and a sound childhood, growing up with my two brothers and my sister. I became a ten-year-old who struggled to decipher English words with help from my mother whose schooling was for eight years at a village school:

> *'Baa, Baa, Black sheep / Have you any wool...'*
>
> 'Amma, *Baa-Baa* is Kannada, not English!'*
>
> 'How true. These English people have lifted words from our language. Never mind, it will be easier to learn.'

This was when we had moved to Delhi, because of my father's job. The mental struggle of transition from speaking Kannada to speaking English and of living and schooling in Delhi served as a springboard for my faculties. Not because English is superior to Kannada in any way but because Delhi of the sixties was a place of great positivity, with a heady mix of cosmopolitan and traditional splendour. Everywhere there was hope and trustfulness in our growth as a nation. It was infectious, and it was the reason I made many of the decisions I did.

As a fifteen-year-old, arms weighed down with books, in

*In Kannada Baa-Baa would mean 'come-come'. It made good sense in the nursery rhyme.

a blue-and-white pinafore, I became too intent on physics, chemistry, hockey and boys from the school across the road. A year later I was the awkward medic, trying too hard for sophistication which side-stepped me through life. And all too soon I was an intern, a surgeon, a wife, a mother, a writer. A woman who got lumped with work, and liked it. I have loved the arduous effort of deep learning, the sheer liveliness of team-work well done, the rapport with communities, the eccentricities and the brave, little-known heroics of people. I have loved the challenge of dangerous tasks and the possibility that I may be able to brighten a small patch of darkness somewhere—if in no other way, then at least as a medical practitioner who knows how powerless one can be sometimes, but who has tried, has always tried…

Destiny takes small steps. It minces along on the balls of its feet as though it will never reach where it must…and *what's this,* my years as a doctor are over. The game is up, I am about to relinquish arms, much like an old farmer who limps away from his rice fields and washes the soft mud clinging to his feet. 'I'm done,' he tells himself, and turns around for a last look. Seeing the weeds and worms, he picks up his arms and heads back.

I too must keep going: there is a clinic that must stay open, there are days to fill and fulfil, absences to endure, meaning to find. Meanwhile, this book.

1

Learning

'Life itself is a slow-burning fire, each cell's carbon turned by oxygen into cooking, sleeping, love-making, stories, laughter, grief.'—Jane Hirshfield; in *Hearth*

Short, plump and dapper in buff-coloured khadi, the health minister surveyed the eager, upturned faces of his audience. Indulging us with a paternal smile, he held forth about the 'cream of the nation' having been chosen to serve suffering humanity in the remote corners of the country.

I was one among fifty medical students who had joined college a week earlier and wearing a sari and heels for the first time. I remember it so well, not because of the extravagant speech I was listening to, but the shared thrill of being a medic and the breathless pleasures it promised. Taking a cue from the seniors, we joked about the minister's speech. Why would we want to be cream, that evil stuff you skimmed off milk? By suffering humanity did he mean sixteen-year-olds in first-time saris that were too tight around the waist and high heels which pinched painfully? As for serving the country, that could wait. The words of the health minister sounded fake then. They would sound fake now.

St John's Medical College (the first Catholic medical college in the world) was founded in 1963 in the city of Bangalore.* There were fifty students to a batch every year, so in comparison to other colleges, it was small. Those were days when the paying of capitation fees to get a seat was unheard of.

My conservative middle-class upbringing did not equip me with any great ambition except that of pleasing those close to me. The novels of A.J. Cronin and perhaps the real-life story of Dr Albert Schweitzer had lured me into medicine. This appeal was heightened by the image of doctors who visited my childhood illnesses. I had come across a copy of *Gray's Anatomy* (my grandfather's) in the attic at home when I was a schoolgirl. The possibility of mastering the complex mysteries of anatomy bewitched me.† More engrossing than *Gray's Anatomy* was an endearing volume, *The Home Doctor*. It explained, with photographs, how the body worked and how common ailments could be treated at home. What kept me rapt was the section on reproductive organs, male and female. I read for the first time about sexual intercourse, pregnancy and reproduction. I understood menstruation. If you know something about the social life of a middle-class girl from a conservative family of the 1960s, you will understand the significance of such knowledge. Of course, I had suspected there was something more to producing babies than the act of exchanging garlands in a marriage. Now I knew.

My parents and others tried gentle persuasion to discourage

---

*The initial funding came from the Catholic community of Germany, anxious after World War II to focus on a positive activity in some part of the under-developed world.

†Years later I found that my grandmother had been tearing off its pages to make paper cones for puffed rice, coconut and jaggery with which she bribed her grandchildren to get chores done. One such task was to catch flies that sailed into the dining room straight from the cattle-shed and to dunk them in a vessel of soapy water. This is what you do: take a bold, open-palm swipe at the said fly or flies and close your palm over the victim with dexterous…that should do.

me from being a doctor. After gaining admission, I listened to their subsequent counsel about selfless service, never working anywhere but in India and definitely marrying some 'very nice chap' from our ilk, with the supreme confidence that I would not fail to fulfil these obligations. How little I knew myself.

The medical college was yet to be built. When I joined, the classes were being held in a two-storeyed rented building in Cooke Town. A thatch-roofed enclosure held together with rugged poles served as the boys' hostel. The boys adjusted rather well, considering that the bamboo hut also housed rats and snakes. Some of the girls were paying guests with neighbouring families. For others there were unused classrooms in a convent school into which three cots, three writing desks, three chairs and three girls were squeezed in. We walked in and out of our rooms clutching our books with great dignity, conscious of being medical students and ever so slightly scornful of the manic little terrors called schoolkids.

With the exception of Lady Harding's in Delhi, medical colleges in India are co-educational. So there came the most dramatic climate change in my life: boys. I had no flair for personal grooming and felt keenly the inadequacy. My mother was a simple, homebound woman. For my splendid foray into college, she packed a medium-sized tin trunk with four sets of skirts with blouses, two saris, underskirts, a night-gown, towels, bedsheets and pillowcases. Wrapped in paper was a clumsy-looking pair of beige-and-gold heeled sandals that she chose for me in Gonicoppal, our local town with five or six shops cosily clustered around the bus stand. Once in college, I realized how ill-equipped I was sartorially and set about embellishing my tin trunk-wardrobe. When my father visited me at the hostel, I sought pocket-money for 'essentials'. A father-daughter equation coloured by mutual shyness meant that he assumed this money was for certain feminine needs and that he should not ask too many questions. I took advantage of his shyness.

My sister, completing her graduation in another college, must have done the same.

Liberties were to be had that were hitherto unthought of. Conveniently distanced from parental control, I traversed new territory, seemingly purposeful but often confused and afraid. I was ignorant of the dangers of those innocent years of early adulthood. But doing well academically was a priority. Many of the faculty at St John's College had given up better-paid jobs in the West and joined the new enterprise. The dissection of bodies, the experiments on frogs to study the neuromuscular systems, the magic of chemistry within body fluids and the marvel of physics that propels a living machine occupied us for three semesters of six months each.

Neat and trim in a medic's coat of white drill, entering the dissection hall for the first time is a moment I will never forget. Long and austere, the sunlit room was adorned with ten long tables topped with stone slabs on which were laid out formalin-soaked cadavers draped in transparent plastic sheets. Five students to a body, a body that would be our companion-plus-silent-teacher for eighteen months. We had each purchased our personal sets of instruments: scalpel, scissors, toothed and non-toothed forceps, a narrow probe and hook; the disarticulated skeleton (costing hundred bucks); and three volumes of *Cunnigham's Dissection Manual*. The professor and his team withstood our shrinking distaste and eased us into work, while the two dissection room flunkeys, not much older than the students, slumped against the doors and sniggered. Mani and Sunder were friendly and actually quite sympathetic. The daily chore of lifting the bodies out of formalin tanks, watching us fumble through the ordeal of cutting into human flesh, lugging the massacred bodies back into the tanks and out again the next day had given them a natural decorum. They knew which group belonged to each body. As for us, the cadaver was all-important. He commanded respect and devotion. We named these primary teachers: Subbu, Charlie, Guru, Swami, Badshah. There was a lone Akkamma assigned to the first batch of five as per alphabetical justice. A feeling of bewilderment about the mystical participation in our lives of these mute figures that once laughed and cried, would come and go. I did not seek answers to such questions.

Bit by painful bit, we got used to smarting eyes, seared throats, smelly hands, the leathery coldness of shrivelled flesh and the malodorous air of death. We plunged beneath skin and fat into muscle, cartilage, nerve and artery. I struggled to adjust, and knew I had done it when one day, halfway through lunch, I realized that I had forgotten to wash my hands. The fingers that held the chapati had just let go off Subbu's armpit…a moment's hesitation, and then I kept on eating.

It is an established routine to begin dissecting the body at the armpit or axilla—the concavity between shoulder and chest—the junction where arm joins trunk. Week after week we cut and probed and worked our way through the upper limb, lower limb, chest, abdomen, pelvis, neck. One among the five in a batch would wield the scalpel while another read out the sequence of dissection from *Cunningham's Manual*.

The professor was a looming figure of a man with an inch-long moustache that seemed to hide the hint of a smile. He had a mercurial temper and could easily reduce me to tears. His mission was to make 'thinking doctors' of every one of us. His passion for anatomy was like that of a fine poet for poetry. He taught us the comparative anatomy of animals, the structure and composition of the variety of cells which constitute an organ, be it liver, skin, bone or brain, the nuanced beauty of creation, its mysteries and evolutionary puzzles. He prodded us to master every detail which is why I was able to retain the knowledge which subsequently made surgery quite simple. Surgery is as much a manual skill as a perfect understanding of structural detail. The usefulness of being able to visualize the contours, size, density and geographical location of every structure is brought home to me each day. The professor made us think. Some of the boys who visited him at home said he served excellent coffee. I found that out much later, in my final year of medical school when I picked up the courage to visit him.

College offered the enchantment of freedom. The mental exertions of study were lightened with recreational activities. There was basketball, throwball, badminton and table tennis for the girls; football, hockey and cricket for the boys. There were movies, cheap restaurants, teenage tattle and the unforgettably sweet boy-girl encounters. Youth is a period when one's absorption with the self can be intense, so focused that it becomes destructive. Friends set you free. Carefree, abrasive, insulting, loving and forever frank, they rescue us from getting swamped in self-importance, or self-pity. I know how much I owe my friends.

Friendships were forged during the long hours in the dissection hall or the physiology lab. We were soon hardened to the horrors of dissection (the worst being the mouth cavity and intestines). Some of the boys resorted to pranks like tying bits of muscle or tendon to dangling plaits or shoving some squidgy bit of anatomy into another's coat pocket. One guy swallowed a piece of muscle for ten bucks! He is now a senior orthopaedic surgeon in the US.

How we talked. What better ambience than that of a formalin-infused room with dead persons revealing their own secrets to fifty would-be doctors on balmy summer mornings in the once-beautiful Bangalore? Who better than seventeen-year-olds to sit in judgment on matters small and big?

There were lectures and slide shows and osteology—the study of bones. A single bone takes a week or two of intense learning during which time it is carried (not without pride) in a commodious all-purpose handbag—the femur, the humerus, scapula or a dainty clavicle nestling between water bottle, lunch box, kerchief, notebooks and pen. Come to think of it, I don't remember boys carrying any such bag. Girls were simply more studious and needed the comfort of proximity with books and bones and other learning aids. When I went home for revision holidays, I took the bones along and made an exhibit of myself, slouched on the sofa or bed leafing through *Gray's Anatomy* while running my fingers over the gently curving pelvic bones. I curled my hair on the clavicle and scratched my neck with the claw-headed ulna. Nobody cared, until the dhobi-woman looking in through the window saw me casually stroking the skull that grinned from my bedside table. She screamed. My mother told me to behave myself.

At college, we continued learning. One day it would be the tracing of the median nerve from upper arm through forearm to its termination in the fingers, another day a dissection of the brachial artery in the cubital fossa. If you accidentally cut a nerve or damaged a blood vessel, your clumsiness was more readily forgiven by the teachers than by your four bench-mates and you suffered, until another disaster happened or an achievement drew praise.

The last few months of learning by dissection were sober and contemplative. We were quieter, less rambunctious, and when we spoke, it was in hushed whispers. The long room with its stone slabs was bleak and empty-looking. Subbu, Badshah, Charles and Akkamma had departed quietly, letting go of upper limb, lower limb, chest, breast, abdomen, perineum, genitals. What remained was the head, or heads—all ten of them resting on cold marble. The mouth cavity with tongue and teeth, the eyes, the ears, the nose. The face represents the person like no other but looking at one's reflection ten, twenty times a day every day will not tell a thing beyond the external. I began to feel a sad, intimate connection with Subbu, having cut into every crevice, fold and fissure of what had been his body.

Drawing the sharp-bladed scalpel over his face was like entering a sanctum unbid. 'Sorry,' I whispered and cut, with as much gentleness as my inexperience allowed. One day we broke into the skull using drills and saws not unlike those of a carpenter. A few weeks of grappling with the bones that make up this cage before cutting through with the gigli saw*: the brain stood grandly alone, delicately shaped, a pale and dirty cream, the lone remnant of a thirty-odd-year-old who had, in death, given himself up to our unknown touch.

*

The department of physiology (the study of how the various organs of the body function) was helmed by a husband-wife pair, reputed internationally for their research in neurophysiology. Guinea pigs, mice, dogs and monkeys were used in the research wing of the department which had a team of assistant staff. We students learnt on frogs. It is easier to dissect a dead human than experiment on a live frog. The first step is to paralyze the slithering amphibian, wriggling wildly in your hand. Nicking the back of the neck dissociates the spinal cord from the brain. This cowardly backstabbing is called *pithing.* The pithed frogs are conscious and breathing and the heart beats dangerously fast beneath your clutching fingers but he will not feel pain when a nerve is stimulated to bring about a specific muscle movement. I found myself unable to handle the animals—I would visualize the frog transformed into a miniature human and fail to complete many of the experiments that every student must do. My hands would tremble, the fingers stiffen and refuse to move over the sliding, skidding, panic-stricken frog. I would feel faint and queasy but told no one how I felt, although a few times a dear friend (bless him!) would do it for me. To this day

---

*A delicate length of wire with metal handles that is draped below a bone like a sling and then slid to and fro, thus cutting with precision.

I recollect the experiments with distaste. Dogs and monkeys were used for more complex experiments on the vital centres of the brain that control breathing and heartbeat. Thankfully the teaching staff took charge of such trials. Students watched. When the usefulness of the animals was over, they were taken away and despatched, painlessly, to their Maker.

I devoured the textbooks of physiology. The best among them were like detective novels in which the reader experiences the thrill of a new curiosity—*what happens?*—and reads on until the mystery is solved. Not just that. A well-written book is a well-written book. Besides knowledge, it brings pure joy. Anatomy and Physiology offer the pure pleasures of learning how human organs are arranged into 'systems'—the respiratory, digestive, cardio-vascular, urinary, neurogenic—which work in synergy with each other to ensure optimal health. No other subject that I learned subsequently came anywhere close to the marvel of learning how the body maintains itself and preserves the miracle of life.

Teaching us the complexities of blood and its components was the associate professor who had a doctorate in haematology from Oxford. Draped in un-ironed kanjeevarams drawn prudishly around her slender frame, this twinkle-eyed blood specialist could take all the ribbing from students while ensuring, *insisting*, on thorough comprehension. Her face took on a special radiance when she explained the mechanism by which this red-coloured substance stays fluid within the body but clots moments after it comes out; how it carries oxygen and nutrients from food to every cell and how it fights the invading armies of disease-producing germs until the battle is won or lost.

Anatomy and physiology, along with pathology and biochemistry, are the cornerstones of medical knowledge. Good teachers, particularly in these basic sciences, are a treasure. The reluctance to share knowledge and skill is perhaps forgivable in matters where profit is the motive. A mithaiwala will keep his recipe for boondi laddus a secret and pass it on to his favourite son. A teacher is not selling laddus. We at St John's were fortunate with our teachers. Some have passed on, and every year, another makes a quiet exit. Among those I met until recently was a handsome couple—she had tutored us in anatomy and he taught us microbiology. The years melted away as we talked of old times. A few of my teachers are still around and occasionally, I get to meet them.

*

In the third year we moved, dutifully, from the dead to the living. There is no irony at all in the fact that we come in through the exit route, first encountering death in the dissection rooms and then entering the hospital wards teeming with life that we must learn to preserve and prolong. None of us stopped to consider the strangeness of moving from the formalin-infused chill of cadavers to the hopeful rows of patients. Armed with the stethoscope and other requisites, I began the third year of my medical life, prodding chests, pummelling bellies, pulling joints and listening with desperate concentration to heart sounds inaudible to my untrained ears. I bolstered my slipping confidence with bravado. It was a pathetic show and I knew it. The bizarre process of being exposed to the myriad wonders of disease and cure was too much, too soon. Ten or more medics would gather around a bed on which lay a man, woman or child—a specimen of medical curiosity that would yield the secrets of a disease. Sympathy? Of course. But *learning*—at the bedside, in the ructions of out-patient clinics, in emergency wards and in the keyed-up sanctity of the operating theatre—was our duty. Even while trudging between wards, getting in the way of doctors, nurses, speeding stretchers, bewildered patients and wailing relatives, we learned how a person falls ill, how the diagnosis is nailed and the treatment decided.

The doctors were busy. They were forever rushing off to the next patient, the next surgery, an emergency, a death, a post-mortem, a meeting, a conference—tackling a capricious mix of censure and acclaim as they went about their duties. In the midst of all this, they had to tutor and instruct students. It is difficult to teach, and tiresome to repeat the lessons to batch after batch of students. Teaching takes time. It brings next to nothing in return. Grade the personality of doctors and you find a curiously speckled range of the meticulous, the arrogant, the showy, the bombastic, the charismatic, the brooding, the mercurial and the quietly efficient. The quality of their instruction is as varied.

Along with the rest, eventually I became bolder and jauntier, moseying into wards with the stethoscope reclining on my neck, coat pockets crammed with the *Hutchinson's Manual of Clinical Medicine*, torch, percussion hammer, tuning fork and scribbled notes. In the evenings I would head back to the hostel with my brain in a whirl. Was this how it was meant to be, this puzzlement and confusion, the wonder and the disenchantment? Was there no easier way of learning to treat the sick? The years in college had done nothing to make me feel for the suffering humanity who I had sworn to serve in my touchingly written essay, a specious masterpiece about selfless service, at the entrance examination. My admiration of all that is noble in medicine got relegated to the out-house of my thoughts. I became more concerned with the reality of night shifts, chaotic clinics and the rough-and-tumble of patient care that would follow me for the rest of my working life. I had moments of deep frustration when I doubted my ability to continue. But studying to be a doctor was my idea, so I had to silence the inner whining and press on.

A doctor posted in the emergency ward told me about his twelve-hour shifts and difficult patients. 'Hardly four hours of sleep in the night,' he griped. 'I survive on coffee…dozens of cups of coffee…' But whenever I went to the cinema with my friends (the movie ticket, dosa and coffee costing two bucks) I saw him in the tortuous queue, nattily dressed, eagerly awaiting his ticket. Seeing me and my friends, he would offer a toothy smile, brush his hair with his fingers, tweak his belt and inch forward with the rest. As did everyone else.

2

'Go West'

It was the summer of 1854. Josiah Grinell, a young man in Washington DC, was dissatisfied with his life. The cautious culture of class and status which pervaded the eastern states of the US, the contempt for physical labour and its covert opposition to liberal values were too stifling for Grinell's enquiring nature. He drifted to New York and there sought the advice of Horace Greeley, the editor of the *New York Herald*. The six words of advice offered by Greeley were: 'Go west, young man. Go west.'

Packing his possessions into a beat-up Land Rover, Grinell drove west until he came to the state of Iowa. The farming community of the region opened his young mind to a new challenge. With the help of three friends, he purchased land and plunged into agriculture. Grinell embraced every hardship and every opportunity. Once he had established himself as a successful farmer, he set up educational and religious institutions. If Iowa has the highest literacy in the US and some of the best public schools and colleges in the country, it is thanks to the enterprising initiative of Josiah Grinell.

I met Grinell in the pages of an essay by Tom Wolfe. In medical college, I too had heard the magic words, 'Go West'. We were envious of the few among us who had a brother or cousin living in utter contentment abroad, as of the handful of our seniors who had moved West and wrote letters in fulsome praise of all things foreign. For lady students, going West came with the rider: *after marriage.* Fortune's favourite girls would always marry doctors working in Britain or the US, discovered for them by aunts and uncles. My family made designs to set up a similar match for me. They found him—a prize catch! I was given the application forms to fill for the ECFMG (Entrance Certificate for Foreign Medical Graduates) examination; I filled it. When the dashing young man visited me in college, I was tongue-tied with shame, for he was such a nice guy and none of it was his fault. Later I picked up courage and wrote him a letter, explaining that my affections lay elsewhere.* He understood, and that was that.

My father†, at that time in Delhi, kept his family at a safe distance from politics and its far-reaching corollaries. I was at home on holiday when the health minister happened to drop by, I think, on an informal visit and I was introduced to him as a final-year medic. 'The United States,' said he. 'That's where you should be! As soon as you graduate, I'll see to it that you're on the plane to New York. And from there…' He rattled off names like Harvard, Stanford, Yale and John Hopkins. Utterly pleased and very flattered, I thanked him profusely. With a few more assurances he drove off and I got a proper dressing down from my father. He cautioned against using 'influence' of any sort to further my career.‡

---

*I had, by then, decided to marry a young man who was a year senior to me in college.

†He joined the freedom struggle when he was nineteen, was jailed three times between 1930 and 1947, and went on to become a Member of the Constituent Assembly, a Member of Parliament and a Union Cabinet Minister.

‡The word 'influence' has long been used in India to mean taking advantage of one's proximity to powerful persons in order to get a job, a seat in a prestigious college, a promotion, a transfer to a workplace of one's liking and so on. This happens in other countries too, and is known as 'a recommendation', or 'putting in a good word'. While this socially accepted gesture of goodwill is

Given a pair of wings and an inbuilt compass, most of us would be up and away, in quest of something better than what is our lot. Dick Whittington walked hundreds of miles to London with its 'streets paved in gold'; Icarus flew towards the golden sun; a decade or so ago, two teenaged Ethiopian boys smuggled themselves aboard an aircraft by clinging to the underside of the wings. Icarus went too close to the sun, burned his wings and fell to earth, the two boys froze to death, but Dick made it big. Travellers, runaway slaves, escaped or banished criminals, invading armies, retreating armies, saints and prophets, traders and tricksters; Ibn Battuta, Marco Polo, Genghis Khan, Taimur, Magellan, Vasco da Gama, Captain Cooke, Nadir Shah, Babur. Migration is the stuff of courage and imagination and has helped speed up human progress. In the 19th century when the newly founded universities of Bombay, Calcutta and Madras Presidencies began to teach English, it brought home the riches of Western thought, and widened the scope of young Indians. Raja Ram Mohan Roy, Sir Syed Khan, C.V. Raman, Rabindranath Tagore, Mahatma Gandhi, Motilal and Jawaharlal Nehru—they went to England to study law, science, mathematics, history, philosophy, literature and medicine. The wealth of knowledge they returned with enriched our country a good deal more than what we lost to the colonial rulers in money and royal treasures.* Families with comfortable means sent their sons to England for higher studies. Along with London-trained barristers of law and Sandhurst-trained defence officers,

---

often genuine and might do no harm, it is more often manipulative, insincere or involves financial and other enticements. It ultimately corrodes society by denying opportunity to deserving persons who do not have 'influence'.

*The exodus of Indians as indentured labour to the sugar plantations of Africa ran parallel to the intellectual drift of educated Indians to the West and was no less important. Their future generations formed the earliest of the Indian diaspora.

were doctors who graduated from London or Edinburgh. (One of my grandfather's brothers was sent to London for medical training but a year later he drowned while swimming in the Thames.) Migration gathered speed after Independence. By the late 1960s, doctors were heading West in droves. The exodus to the Middle East, particularly from Kerala, began two decades later.

I remember myself as a serious, secretly ambitious and confused young woman. I succumbed to infatuations and giddy romance before finding myself seriously, enchantedly in love. I tussled with parental control. But somehow, in the midst of my emotional turmoil, I remained focused on my medical training. The glimmer of a sense of purpose came in my final year when the simple lucidity and beauty of surgical knowledge and technique awakened a new-found gladness. I call it gladness because learning gives me more pleasure than almost any other venue of joy. Dr M.V. Bansod, our professor, was one of those rare surgeons with a genuine concern for the future of his students. He had a marvellous way of driving home the essence of *chirugia*: a narrowed tube? Dilate it. Blocked gut? Unblock it. Tumour? Excise! Dead tissue? Cut it out! Broken bone? Fix it! The practical, direct principles of surgery delighted me, just as the act of repairing a broken toy delights a child.

Surgery is an ancient skill. Egyptian mummies have been found with artificial teeth and well-set fractures; trepanning—drilling a hole in the skull to give the evil spirit causing disease a way out—was practised 5000 years ago. Neurosurgeons use the same technique to lessen the pressure within the skull to save accident victims from dying of serious head injuries. In Rome, records of good surgical practice exist from the 1st century CE. Celsus wrote about the need to ensure cleanliness, the washing of wounds in sugar and thyme oil which deaden pain, and the use of ligatures for arterial bleeding. His comments on the qualities of a surgeon are astute:

> A surgeon should be youthful or at any rate nearer youth than age; with a strong and steady hand which never trembles, and ready to use the left hand as well as the right; with vision sharp and clear, spirit undaunted; filled with pity, so that he wishes to cure his patient, yet is not moved by his cries, to go too fast, or cut less than necessary; but he does everything just as if the cries of pain cause him no emotion.

In the final year at college, I won a coveted prize in surgery and thought maybe I could be a surgeon. One of the physicians who often pronounced withering comments about the rudely physical nature of surgery as opposed to the intellectual depth of medicine said, mockingly: 'I see that you prefer to be a gross surgeon and not a clever physician.'

'Yes, sir,' I replied.

I stayed firm in my resolve. Self-belief and stubbornness—my tattered graces—sustained me, until a year later, a rare opportunity came my way.

*

The UK and the US remain the two most attractive countries for Indian doctors seeking better prospects. You cannot throw a stethoscope (or a knee hammer if you want a victim) in either country without hitting one of our doctors. During a three-month writing fellowship in Iowa some years ago, I spoke at a gathering of Indian physicians in a small town on the west coast. The venue, a doctor's home, was opulent: a winding bannistered staircase, pillars rising out of carved lotuses, Kashmiri carpets, a profusely ornamental garden and a swimming pool with stylized figurines looking on. My wonderment was akin to what I experience when watching certain Hindi films. But in all truth, I have met many more Indian doctors known for their skills rather than the sumptuousness of their lifestyle.*

Contrast the circumstances of expatriate doctors with those of doctors who could not go or chose not to. I recall the rueful gripes of a dear person who had set his heart on neurosurgery and was able to get a junior post at BYL Nair Hospital in Bombay. He was elated to be able to work with Dr VG Daftary, one of the pioneers of brain surgery in the country. He did not want to trade it for anything. It had its good moments, great moments, but it was just too much work. 'The six hundred I earn barely cover my expenses,' he said. 'I share a room with three others. We chafe against each other all the time.' The doctors, nurses and other staff were overworked and underpaid. Frayed tempers, backbiting and meanness were part of the job. He withstood it for a year. When he could not get one of the two post-graduate seats which came up, he applied for a work permit in the UK, joined there as a casualty medical officer and worked his way up.

To understand why doctors leave the country, we must head back to pre-Independent India. Soon after the ravages of Bengal by the famine of 1942 (when an estimated 20 to 30 lakh people died due to starvation, disease and poor food distribution), the government set up a committee to devise a plan for improving the welfare system. It was headed by Sir Joseph Bhore, of the Indian Civil Service. The final report of the Bhore Committee made in 1946 was introduced thus:

> If it were possible to evaluate the loss, which this country annually suffers through the avoidable waste of valuable

*The leakage of young graduates to the West is common to several countries in the subcontinent. A few years ago I was in Karachi for two weeks, for a literary project. I asked if I could visit some of their medical centres and was able to see the Aga Khan Hospital and the Sind Institute of Urology and Transplantation. The specialist doctors were almost all trained in the US or the UK and had chosen to return. Given the unpredictable environment in the country, this surprised me. I asked, and a surgeon told me: 'There are two types of migrations from

> human material and the lowering of human efficiency through malnutrition and preventable morbidity, we feel that the result would be so startling that the whole country would be aroused and would not rest until a radical change had been brought about.

The guidelines were succinct: A state-run, decentralized, tiered health-care system that would reach the 'the tillers of the soil' in the villages; the integration of preventive and curative services; the development of Primary Health Centres, one per 40,000 people, with a thirty-bedded hospital and two doctors; and major changes in medical education, including three months of training in preventive and social medicine.

In the early years following Independence, hospitals, health centres and sub-centres were built in accordance with the proposal. Doctors, nurses and health workers were sent to small towns and villages. A sound welfare system seemed altogether possible, thanks largely to some of the finest men and women in the profession, like Dr Sushila Nayyar and Dr B.C. Roy who were instrumental in ensuring its success.

In the 1960s and early '70s, everyone went to government hospitals and it was normal for families to visit an ailing relative or friend in clean, well-maintained wards. I remember the birth of my younger brother at the government hospital in Madikeri (a town in Kodagu district, Karnataka), its antiseptic corridors, the nurses in white, the red hospital blanket beneath which lay my mother and the little thing she had just delivered. A year or so later, I was there with a piece of glass embedded in my heel; my brother was taken to the same hospital with a fish bone

---

our country and yours. One is in search of livelihood due to severe economic distress. The other, as with doctors, is to improve our academic (and material) prospects. It is our duty to come back. But most of us do not have the resilience it takes…' I talked to several others who were keeping their options open. If the safety levels in the country deteriorated to critical levels, they would go back to the West.

stuck in his throat and my sister with an abscess in her leg. It was one of the two hospitals in our district and there was little cause for complaint.

In 1951, the population of India was 33 crores, with an average life expectancy of thirty-two years. A mere 18 per cent of Indians were literate. In 1971, the population stood at 56 crores, that is, an increase of 10 crore people in each of the two preceding decades, or 1 crore every year. Life expectancy had improved to forty-eight years. Independent India was healthier by far when compared to British India. Social, economic and welfare factors reduced the risks of early death. Better nutrition, housing, education and government-funded health care (with immunizations, care of pregnant women and the newborn, effective treatment of dangerous communicable diseases) ensured that a grandparent was not a mere faded photograph, framed and hung on the wall.

However, meeting the needs of a rapidly growing population posed problems. The training of doctors in medical colleges is highly subsidised. MBBS stands for Bachelor of Medicine and Bachelor of Surgery, so in effect the degree-holder is a doctor in the complete sense of the term—she is qualified to treat common medical and surgical problems. Nine out of ten patients who visit a general hospital can be treated by doctors who have an MBBS degree while one might need a specialist opinion. However in reality, these hospitals refuse to take on the simplest of challenges, and hastily bundle patients off to higher centres.*

So here we are in 2021, nowhere near ensuring basic health care for our citizens. Eighty per cent of hospital beds are in the cities while 70 per cent of our people live in semi-urban and rural areas. Seventy crore people (more than ten times

*This is not always the case. A significant number of doctors have worked within the government system with great dedication and created centres of excellence in India.

the population of UK or twice that of US and Canada put together) get unsatisfactory treatment or none.

It is important to look at the problem from every angle: the government which claims to have equipped and staffed the hospitals does nothing to ensure that the system works. The peripheral hospitals are inadequately staffed and equipped; corruption and the rampant misuse of funds is common; doctors sent to the small towns and villages either pull strings to get better placements or languish at their jobs, lazy and inefficient. They turn out to be as covetous and grasping as any babu in a government office. The public does not protest. The doctors absent themselves from official duty and work privately, while earning salary plus perks from the government. Many claim to have paid bribes to higher officials in order to get the jobs in government; they are pliant enough to work within a corrupt system and readily adjust to the unethical conduct of their peers. Rural work in government hospitals is very difficult because of this ingrained tendency for malpractice. I had a taste of it during my internship and it definitely turned me off.

City practice, on the other hand, demands specialization. The medical curriculum in India, although based on the Western medical system, is unable to keep pace with specialized study and research that are essential. This has led to frustration among doctors keen to pursue academic excellence. Postgraduate seats are inadequate; bribe money—presently amounting to a crore of rupees or more—is often essential for the college gates to open. Given these realities, what do bright, ambitious young graduates do but beat it West as soon as they possibly can? If the motherland does not offer the means to realize your dreams, you seek a better surrogate.

Doctors who go abroad put in years of hard work under intense pressure; and the rewards are handsome. The government hopes to entice them back with facile adulation during the Pravasi Bharatiya Diwas (a day which celebrates the contribution of Overseas Indians to the country), celebrated with much publicity for over a decade. The non-resident Indian doctors arrive in droves and proclaim dreams of starting centres of excellence in India. The government is elated and repeats its artful attempts to woo them back. It doesn't work. For those accustomed to the professional standards of the West, it is near impossible to work within India's crooked system. One can say that fraudulence is universal but nowhere is it as pervasive and accepted as in our motherland. No matter how much we wish to glorify our ancient cultures and religious fixations, we have no cause to congratulate ourselves as the keepers of people's health. The recognition the immigrant doctors receive in the country of their choice is richly deserved. They will come when they have retired from their jobs in the West, if they come at all. Let's not grudge them joy in retirement. The fact remains, that for medical welfare in India, the vacuum left behind by them is a tragedy.

Immigrant Indians have not remained insensitive to the problems in their country of birth. The money and gifts we receive from our expatriate countrymen run into millions of dollars. While some prefer to concentrate exclusively on family, others donate to political parties or to charity. They have gifted the country pockets of affluence in parts of Punjab, Kerala, Andhra Pradesh and Gujarat. All this means that future generations too are propelled to the West.

A smaller, more committed fraction of our expatriate countrymen channel generous amounts of money for urgently needed medical resources, having first ensured the genuineness of the cause. Until a few years ago, expatriate doctors were earnestly donating equipment (ultrasound machines, foetal dopplers, disposable catheters, suture material) to our hospitals, spending time and effort to ensure that the gifts reached their destinations. Servicing these gadgets is problematic, expensive or impossible. But we, the Bharatvasis, are attracted to all things foreign and free.*

*

When I finished college, what I had were the stethoscope, the MBBS certificate and the miles and miles of knowledge written into the sulci and gyri of my brain. Although I never truly acquired any other form of sophistication, I found I had acquired a certain level of maturity in my understanding of science. The company of batchmates all similarly flapping in unknown waters, trying to learn the game of survival made it a little bit easier. Most of us stayed afloat.

*At a hospital in Uttar Pradesh where I worked, we received consignments of disposable items from the UK. A lot of it was put to good use, at a time when medical technology in India was in its infancy and we relied heavily on foreign-made goods. This changed about two decades ago, with the manufacture of indigenous, quality medical products. It is therefore better to give (and accept) help in the form of money sent through recognized channels for the purchase of locally available equipment.

3

Internship

'One of the first duties of the physician is to educate the masses not to take medicine.'—Sir William Osler in *Aphorisms from his Bedside Teachings.*

I saw Sivaji Ganesan in *Veerapandian Kattabomman* (the film on the life of an 18th-century Tamil chieftain of lore) and acquired the first of my film heroes. Tamil films were the rage, those days. (The film *Gunasundari* mesmerised with the coquetry of svelte Padmini and a cutely caked-up Gemini Ganesan; and what would I not give to watch Nagesh once more as *Server Sunderam?)*

My taste in films is of no significance except that it began with my first unforgettable visit to a city when I was seven or eight. It took half a day in our Standard Vanguard to cover the 70-odd kilometres from our home in Kodagu to Mysore, a magic-land of palace, cinema, zoo, circus, and brahmin lunch homes. We ate belly-pleasing fare sitting cross-legged in the long dining hall of Modern Hindu Hotel—a rupee a meal. At another, more stylish place I swallowed my first spoon of ice cream and hated it. (I have since learned to eat unlimited amounts, much to the dismay of he who pays.) I love being in a city, knowing I don't have to live there.

Having finished college, I found myself unhappy in a vague sort of way. My personal life was tangled and my parents were anxious to whisk me off to safer pastures. So, for my internship, I was enrolled at the government hospital in Mysore. The city exemplifies dignified grandeur and serenity, its past glory dissolving at an unhurried pace while modernity takes over, bit by bit. No matter where you go, the palace is never more than a few minutes away. Until twenty years ago, the residential parts of Mysore displayed a traditional reticence—modest tile-roofed homes from which issued the muted notes of Carnatic music. In one such neighbourhood, my parents rented a house for a year while I completed my internship.

The Krishna Rajendra Hospital and Medical College were built in the latter part of the 19th century when Mysore was ruled by the Wodeyar royals. K.R. Hospital is in the heart of the city between the market and the vast palace properties. Its architecture resonates with that of the palace while escaping the puzzling mix of English, French and Byzantine craftsmanship on view at the imperial abode of the Mysore kings.

It was a dog's life—internship; a penalty year of aching legs, sleep-deprivation, irritability, hunger pangs and the anxieties of ignorance. The intern was at the receiving end of everybody's frustration: patients emptied their store of invective on us, nurses snapped and doctors blamed the despairing novice for every glitch. Internship takes you through Medicine, Surgery and Gynaecology, with shorter stints in some of the specialities like the eye, skin, bone and mind departments, and three months of rural work. I started with Medicine in Unit One. It was headed by Professor K.G. Das, whose diagnostic skills were the finest and his concern for his patients, real. He went about his ward rounds without haste, taking time to demonstrate clinical signs and explain the treatment for each illness to medical students and interns. Thereafter, the hectic demands of the out-patient clinic occupied him till late afternoon.

The next in hierarchy was the ever-smiling associate professor who treated his junior staff to a coffee session in the canteen after the rounds. He was genial and chatty. His main concerns were the blunder and folly of other doctors. Not wanting to miss the coffee and a chance to rest our feet, we went every day, and amidst a dense fog of cigarette smoke, listened.

On certain days when the professor was held up at a meeting, this same associate professor took charge. He was casual about discipline and finished the rounds in less than an hour, which was most agreeable. But he treated the nurses and general-ward patients with contempt. One afternoon during a tutorial for fourth-year medics, he instructed a student to examine a young man admitted with a birth defect in the heart. When she had finished, he said, 'He has a lump in his groin. Check it.' The girl was hesitant and the patient clearly unhappy.* For a young man to lower his trousers and permit a young woman to check a lump in the groin with others looking on was difficult. He pleaded with his eyes. 'Come on, we don't have all day,' snapped the doctor with a nasty gleam in his eyes. The young man undressed, stretched out on the bed and averted his eyes. It was no less difficult for the medic who was near tears by the time she finished. When the patient got up and pulled up his trousers, the doctor reached out to pat his shoulder. The patient shrugged off the patronizing gesture and turned away. We proceeded to the next bed.

The male and the female medical wards were where I spent most of the next three months, admitting and treating patients, performing minor procedures like removing fluid collected in the chest or belly—due to tuberculosis, cancer or liver disease—cleaning bedsores, introducing catheters, draining hydroceles.

---

*The unwritten rule is that general-ward patients allow physical examination by students. If a clinical condition is interesting, the sufferer is presented to the entire batch. He cannot refuse, since the hospital stay with the treatment—which really amounts to a bed, food, aspirin and rudeness—are free.

The wards filled up quickly and by evening it was two-to-a-bed and then the floor.

On any normal day I had fifteen to twenty injections to give and some of them, twice a day. Syringes (of 2-, 5- and 10-ml capacity) boiled in a foot-long sterilizer in which floated needles of various sizes. It was a cramped room where nurses kept their registers, keys, tiffin boxes, purses, umbrellas; not uncommonly, there would be a live impediment in the form of a child (of one of the nurses). We managed. In one corner on the wall hung bunches of keys to a couple of lockers in which morphine, pethidine, barbiturates and largactyl were stored, and made accessible only to the senior nursing staff. What I remember is the constant flurry of interns squeezing our way in and out holding loaded syringes. There were long moments of frustration, waiting for a syringe or pleading with the in-charge nurse for a new needle, the older ones being disfigured and blunted from repeated use on squirming patients. I tried every trick to reach the sterilizer before a fellow-intern grabbed the syringe or needle of the desired size, in which case it meant waiting until it was boiled again. On my list of patients was a young boy who was prescribed twice-daily penicillin shots. One evening when I approached him with the thickly white liquid loaded in a syringe, he said: 'Akka, you hurt me too much. I want someone else to give it.'

'Not my fault, the needle is blunt,' I snapped. 'Just turn round…'

He curled his emaciated body into position. His shoulders shook.

'It won't hurt much, I promise.'

Every time I approached him, I felt I was indulging in a criminal act.

Three months later, I moved from the medical wards to the surgical. A surgical intern's task is to get the patients ready for surgery, and to assist in the operating theatre, besides doing ward work. Watching the surgeons in the OT, my hands itched. The Professor of Surgery was unsparing in his criticism. We grumbled bitterly about his strictness but admired his dexterity. My first surgical feat was less than grand. I lanced an abscess. Gloating all the way in the bus home, I announced my triumph at home, highlighting the location and size of the abscess, and smell of the pus which filled three kidney trays. My mother grabbed the tumbler of coffee from my hands and chased me off for a bath. Thereafter every evening, I had to make an inglorious entry through the back door, bathe and change my clothes before I could eat or drink.

Months sped by. The wards sobbed with a multitude of agonies and I struggled to match my inadequate skills with required competence. In the midst of all the negatives and many positives of a working day, I reaffirmed my love of surgery. I was going to be a surgeon. Was it the practical nature of surgery which attracted me, or was it the theatrical?

Internship brought home the truth about our welfare system. A doctor can be judged as good, not-so-good or mediocre. The most dangerous is the unprincipled doctor whose crookedness is intentional and does not easily lend itself to amendment. This makes for a variety of ways by which patients are harmed and the profession sullied. At K.R. Hospital there was one doctor who got away with doing nothing except appear and disappear from the wards just as he pleased, twirling the key to his lemon-green Bajaj Super in one hand and smiling at no one in particular. He should have been pulled up, but the fact that he was the nephew of some local politician meant that no one dared to. Another rotund, rather stupid-looking man abased himself before his seniors by offering to buy their vegetables, carry their umbrellas and briefcases. When the seniors were not around, he was crude and sarcastic. I wonder what happened to these doctors and to their patients in their several decades of practice.

And there was Dr Narendra: disciplined, untiring, infatuated with work and anxious to exhibit his work, a duty-machine that could not switch off. His work itself was exemplary but he did not appeal to me very much. In the evenings, Dr Narendra was in charge. One day when we had finished work for the day, I told him that a patient had approached me with money. I declined, and reassured her that we were paid for our work. She looked at me with puzzlement. Tucking the envelope away, she pulled out another. 'This is for sir. Please give it.' she meant Dr Narendra who had operated on her. 'Put it away,' I said. 'He will not be pleased.'

He was certainly not pleased—with me. His ever-cheerful face became expressionless. 'Don't ever do that again,' he told me. 'Patients offer money as a mark of gratitude. It is an insult to the giver to refuse the money. Once a villager brought me rupee notes in a bucket. A bucketful of notes, can you imagine? He was saying thank you, like this woman who offered the envelope. You must not refuse a thank you.'

There are many ways of duping the gullible. For instance, the hospital pharmacy was forever out-of-stock for most medicines except aspirin, iron and cheap vitamin tablets doled out in the general wards like chaff: one black, one white and one yellow pill were dribbled off a bottle into obediently cupped palms by a junior nurse or an ayah. 'Akka… they don't work.' Of course they don't. Antibiotics, cough syrups, and injection vials marked '*Government Property. Not for Sale*' found their way mysteriously into medical shops across the road. Patients who should have got these drugs free had to buy them, as special medicines. Every day, somewhere in the hospital there would be a ruckus, with a patient demanding better medicines or service. Always he was shouted down.

None of the doctors complained. I didn't either. I persuaded myself that I was too junior to meddle in such business, and meekly did my duty. Silence in the face of serious wrong is diluted morality, cowardly and dishonest; to decry it years later is a futile squeal of self-endorsement: see, *my* hands are clean. Our silence allowed malpractice to become entrenched within the system. Somewhere along the way I started to speak up. Each time I was met by icy silence and a swift change of topic.

During my internship, a surgeon was appointed at the newly established cardio-thoracic department. He had returned four weeks earlier after specialist training in the UK. After being assigned a couple of newly painted rooms, a few pieces of equipment and a clueless ward boy, he was asked to set up post-graduate studies in thoracic surgery. My memory is of a tall, personable surgeon, moving about the hospital bemused and lost, like the party-guest who has little in common with any of the others. I would sometimes meet his wife on the bus—on her way to the market to buy some vegetables, she would say. I remember feeling surprised, for my image of a woman just returned from abroad was different.

One afternoon, reading up some technical details in the hospital library, I picked up courage to speak to this foreign-returned Chest Surgeon. What was it like to be back in India?

'I like it well enough,' he said. 'My wife's from Mysore, I'm from Gwalior. We had decided to come back and it was a toss-up between my place and hers. She won.'

I wanted to know how the hospital compared with those in Britain.

'What can I say? I haven't done any work in all these three weeks. The few patients I've seen need to be worked up in detail. Some need surgery. I require staff, materials, medicines. Every day I'm told this or that will be done, but nothing happens.' He had been excited by the prospect of setting up a cardio-thoracic unit in Mysore and had quit his senior job at the University of Leeds.

'Have you seen a cardiac or lung surgery?' he asked. I hadn't. 'When you're operating within the chest cavity, the movements of the lung (which inflates and deflates with every breath) can interfere with your field of work. The anaesthetist uses a double-lumen tube (one branch going into each lung) to deliver the anaesthetic gases which keep the patient asleep during surgery.' He made a sketch on his notepad. 'This way, one lung can be kept inflated and the other kept empty, like a shrunken balloon, so it does not clutter the operating field.

'We need trained nurses and a technician to see that every piece of equipment is in working condition; a lab that can check arterial blood gases during and soon after surgery; an Intensive Care Unit. I wish they had appointed me after putting together these basics.' He said he was unhappy to earn for nothing.

Over the next few months, I was to see his dismal figure in his office or in the library. Subsequently there came a change, a spring in his step, and activity in the hospital wing that had been marked for the ICU. The very first thoracic case was to happen that week. The surgeon had approached a thoracic specialist in Bangalore and with his help, gathered a trained team and an anaesthetist. A week later the hospital was abuzz with the news that the surgeon had opened the chest cavity and excised a tumour. The patient was doing fine.

I have often wondered what would have happened if this surgeon had given up and gone back to England.

It takes just one person to initiate a change.

4

Truly Rural

The last three months of internship were reserved for rural posting, in the neighbouring district of Mandya. The town is a short journey by train from Mysore. It had begun to assert itself as the district headquarters, and sported a railway station, a neat and salubrious park, a cinema house, a few 'Tiffin Homes' and the district hospital. The hour-long journey by train took us to Mandya where we had enough time to partake of coffee and bondas before heading for the hospital to wait for the medical officer. The kind gentleman spoke to us, for twenty to thirty minutes, about our work during the rural stint. Then the attendance register was passed around for signatures after which we were let off. What remained of the day was spent eating lunch and dawdling in the park till late afternoon when we boarded the train back to Mysore. I was home by 6 p.m., visibly fatigued after a day's work.

It was all very pleasing: tense nerves unjangled! We arranged a few picnics from Mandya, thanks to the benevolence of the medical officer. Twice, he organized village visits. We went in a health-department jeep to a clutch of hamlets 16 kilometres away and advised bewildered women about nutritious food. We questioned them on their views about family planning. 'It is unwise to have more than two,' said we. They listened gravely. We did not see young women and asked where they were. They were washing clothes at the pond, herding goats, pounding grain. The children were in school, we were told, but many who hung about the huts were of schoolgoing age.

Of the few things I remember about those three months is the curiosity and kindness of the villagers, the chatty women, the shy women, and the starkness of their lives. The district officer talked, the village elder talked. The women served refreshments and sent us on our way. Once when we headed for the jeep, a young lad came alongside, eager to talk. We were as awkward as he, and nudged each other to say something.

'Have you finished school?' asked Vasanthi, one of the interns.

'Seventh pass. I can write little, read little.' Then he blurted out, 'I'm to get married.'

'You're too young!'

'How old *are* you?'

'My mother says I'm old enough to bring home a daughter-in-law. My four brothers and two sisters are married. My brothers' wives need help with the firewood and the threshing.' The girl was from Panchavalli. 'Big people. Tobacco-growing,' he added, with the hint of a smirk on his boyish face. The wedding was to take place in early summer. 'Akka…how to…how to…not have more than two?'

Advice was given and listened to. Explaining contraception to a young man was challenging but Vasanthi managed. She explained the rhythm-method, with dates, on a piece of paper. He invited us to his wedding and went away satisfied. Was he able to limit his offspring? We would never know.

The highlight of my rural stint was a sterilization camp held in a village near Mandya. Three doctors, with the assistance of three interns, were to operate on forty women picked from a cluster of villages. On a sultry May morning we set out in two jeeps. I constricted myself into available space at the back of one, with two nurses in starched white saris, an ayah of vigorous dimensions, a ward-boy, cartons of medicines, drip stands, bottles, basins and bedpans. We jolted over mud roads, the wheels raising reckless clouds of dust, much to our breathing discomfort. The jeep pulled up on an arid field where two men were at work, rigging a stretch of tarpaulin held aloft on poles: the operating theatre.

Coffee and snacks first; then work. The doctors bantered with the nurses who unpacked instruments and readied the stage. The ward-boy whistled and the ayah ushered the waiting women into the tent, smiling kindly. A corner was screened off with sheets. Minutes later, a row of terrified-looking women in their twenties and thirties, emerged in underskirt and blouse, having shed their saris behind the screen. A woman with a long, pinched face and a red bindi was led to one of the three stretchers sent the previous day from the district hospital. The lady doctor donned a mask, and an ill-fitting cap which did little to cover her curly hair. She instructed the woman to climb on to the table and then stuck a needle in her wrist to set up a drip. She washed her hands at a basin resting on a stool, with me pouring water from a mug. Pulling on a pair of operating gloves, she swabbed the lower part of the patient's belly with an antiseptic and injected a local anaesthetic into the incision-site. 'Must finish all the cases by four,' she muttered, picking up the scalpel. As she cut, the patient let out a scream and wriggled out of her reach, dislodging the intravenous drip. The ward-boy pinned her by the shoulders, I held on to her legs while the ayah stuck the needle back into the wrist. The doctor pressed on. She had twelve more cases to finish by four, what did this woman think, was she special?

'Have you not given birth? Was that not painful?'

On two of the three operating tables the scene repeated itself, creating various degrees of pandemonium. The third went quietly about his work. He was competent and kind and as it usually happens, so was his team. I saw the ayah slap a few women who proved to be difficult. Seven of the waiting quarry grabbed their clothes and bolted, a humdrum pre-operative complication, given the situation. The remaining women hung on with stoic calm, concealing fear with the edge of their saris held over their mouths. Not one of the village spectators protested against the barbarity conducted before their eyes on their women.

The Indian male is terrified of the sterilization procedure (which is simpler for men) but he expects the woman to endure it nonetheless. Nothing has changed since. A few big companies have a scheme whereby a male employee who volunteers for sterilization gets a salary hike. I know only one brave guy, a 'hero', who chose to make use of this scheme, had one child, a girl who is now an engineer. The company he worked for gave him a salary hike for having the surgery. The fear of sterilization is not the fault of men, poor things. They are the weaker sex.

I remember coming home after that sterilization camp. I bunked duty for several days, anguishing over my own future, resolving never to be a doctor like the two I witnessed that day. What sort of doctor *would* I be? I was losing my grip. My personal life was stationary, thanks to the many restrictions imposed by my parents. It occurs all the time, in every community and class. Parents cannot conceive that children have dreams of their own, and that some children are wired differently. The astrologer who forecast my future years back was right about one thing: I would have a difficult life. Would it also be beautiful? I would find out.

In that year of internship, although enfolded in the security of family affections, I was solitary and alone. Fervently seeking my selfhood, I wavered and failed and tried again. My stronger self tussled with my weaker self which was tempted to follow tradition, please my family, be spoken well of, besides being assured of lifelong security. I have since understood that members of a family—even those brought up with conservative

Indian values—love and respect each when each is allowed the freedom to live and grow in her way. The forced hand of parental control does not work. Ever.

I was learning, slowly and painfully, to think for myself. I had begun to defy parental control from my late medical college years but most of that was instinctive and somewhat selfish. How was a young woman to break free of age-old control systems and define her own life? If she deprives herself of the rudder of parental care, she must either reach for other means of support, or swim free. Some of the books that I was reading during that time must have helped. Among them were collected essays of Emerson, works of Thoreau and Tagore, Gandhi's *My Experiments with Truth*, Pasternak's *Dr Zhivago* and Maugham's *Of Human Bondage.* Indeed, reading became my ultimate stimulant. I became more aware of myself and my deficiencies. In moments of despair, I walked from the hospital in the direction of our home which was five kilometres away. There was a school for deaf and dumb children along the way which I was curious about. After walking past it a few times, I went up the many steps made of unevenly laid bricks into the office of the headmistress. I said something about the purpose of my visit, realizing as I spoke, that I wasn't making much sense. 'I thought I'd meet some children. I could do something for them, maybe. Teeth…feet…you know, any problems…' I mumbled foolishly.

She summoned a group of students who were at work in the garden. 'This doctor has come all the way from the big hospital. Why don't you show her what you're doing?' They led me to the back of the building where on a diligently tended plot measuring about ten-by-five paces, orange-red marigold and delicate pink dahlia grew along with tomato, brinjal and bhindi. I questioned them with hand gestures: how come? Should each variety of flower and vegetable not be on a separate plot? They giggled, punched and shoved each other and smiled mischievously at me. They shook their heads: no, no. Back in the office, the headmistress explained how a local farmer who came to admit his son at the school had shown them that a mixing of varieties yielded healthier plants, just like inter-community marriages yield more robust children. He was proved right. They grow a rich yield of vegetables and a colourful range of flowers all through the year. I have since used this method in our garden.

I was served coffee and kodubale. The headmistress asked me if I could spare the time to do a health check-up for the students. 'It will be a big help,' she said. I felt flattered. Being in need of help myself, I wanted to help. Equipped with a first-aid kit and medicines put together by a nurse who was my friend, I went. Over three Sunday afternoons, I examined the children, assiduously measuring height and weight, checking teeth and tonsil, chest, belly, eye, hair and skin. I filled a notebook with details of my diagnosis proclaimed in capital letters: DENTAL CARIES. HOOKWORM. ANAEMIA. FURUNCULOSIS. MYOPIA.

They were healthy kids, most of them, and lots of fun. I was rewarded with bananas and apples. Walking home from the bus stop I heard a juvenile, soulful rendering of 'Himagiri Thanaye' floating from one of the houses where music was being taught. Smiling, I went home. 'You look happy,' my mother observed. 'Must have been an easy day.'

The three months of rural work was to end with a week's intensive training in Kollegal. We would live among the villagers and learn valuable lessons about their health and living conditions. From the seniors who had finished the posting, we knew that the interns stayed in a women's hostel in the town of Kollegal (well-removed from a rural society), ate at local restaurants, saw a movie or two and made a few visits to a village as and when it pleased the medical officer. Excellent. It would be an agreeable break. We made plans to include a picnic in the week's activities. Two days before the scheduled week it dawned on me that I wasn't enthusiastic about the farce and pleaded with the medical officer, offering some spurious excuse to be let off. I did not feel any guilt.

The internship was coming to an end. The seniors organized a farewell tea with masala dosa, kesari baath and coffee. After which they breathed deeply and prepared themselves for the next batch of beginners.

5

Bones

Unable to progress in my personal or professional life, I took the job of a senior house surgeon in orthopaedics. The chance to learn the precision of mending broken bones from Dr Gyanchand was my good fortune, even though it was without a salary. He was among the best of teachers, a winsome man—short of stature, magnetic eyed and stocky, with a dry tuneful voice which adapted itself to English, Kannada or the hybridized Hindi of Mysore. When he picked up the knife, he was all grace and skill. From him more than any other, I learnt how surgery must be done.

His instinctive ability to pin down the diagnosis of the most intractable illness brought patients in droves. His treatment—be it surgery, Plaster-of-Paris-immobilization, exercises or medicine—was simple, quick and inexpensive. You could be fooled into thinking it was easy. In his work, there was none of the hesitation, doubling-back, cautionary checks, the flutter or the fuss of excess which mar the clean beauty of surgical technique and diminish the outcome. A couple of times every week, after his work at the hospital, Dr Gyanchand would drive his commodious Standard Vanguard through the palace gates to check on the most elite of his patients: Jayachamarajendra Wodeyar, the erstwhile Maharaja of Mysore who later became the governor of Tamil Nadu. A severe diabetic, he was suffering from early gangrenous changes in his foot.

A fractured bone is the most common ailment that brings a patient to the orthopaedic surgeon.* Following the morning ward rounds I would go to the outpatient department where half a dozen patients waited on the bench outside the door, each supporting an arm, a wrist, leg or ankle, with, sometimes, a wife or mother to help. My job was to arrange for X-rays and then assist the boss in fixing the broken bone. We used the 'drip method' of anaesthesia, with ether—a safe, short-term anaesthetic. I would hold the wired, gauze-covered mask over the patient's face and dribble liquid ether from a dark brown bottle over the mask. The room would fill with the sweet smell of vaporizing ether well before the patient drifted into sleep.

'Hold the jaw up, or the tongue will fall back and obstruct breathing,' the boss would say as he gauged the position of the fragmented bone on the X-ray and walked his fingers over the misshapen contours of the limb. He would stand facing the patient, take the affected arm by the hand as if in greeting and pull steadily, with the ward boy gripping the arm at the elbow and applying counter-traction. Within seconds the bones would click audibly into place. I would take off the ether-mask, ensure that the patient's breathing was even and then go round the stretcher to steady the arm while the boss applied wet sheets of Plaster of Paris in a cylinder around the wrist and forearm. I would hold the position until the plaster hardened and set, stabilizing the bone. A few minutes later the patient, dazed and unsteady, would join the rest on the same 'pre and post-op' bench.

---

*The word ortho-paedic means straight-child and originated from the manoeuvres used to correct bone deformities in children. In untreated fractures, the broken ends of a bone join without alignment, leading to deformities. Many a child who broke a bone in the days of yore lived the rest of her life with a grossly misshapen limb, the broken ends having fused together over time but without being set in the proper position. A bone doctor straightens the broken ends and fits them back into place.

Work spilled over from one action-packed day to the next. Operating days were frenetic, with delays, lack of available operating theatres, shortage of anaesthetists, nurses and medicines. Patients in need of surgery underwent the pre-operative preparation of shaving the affected area the evening before. Early next morning after a bath (and sometimes an enema), they were dressed in shapeless hospital gowns fastened along the back with a snarl of tapes and strings, a few of which were always missing. In this ungainly attire they waited, with nothing to eat or drink, sometimes till 1 p.m. or after, either to be wheeled into the theatre or to be told sorry, next time. Surgeries went on till late evening, until the list was exhausted or a serious emergency took precedence over the rest. General-ward patients were the enduring veterans of many cancellations.

Work went smoothly, my personal life did not. Tussling with the family can be enervating, all that hurt and anger directed at those we love, is so pointless. I often doubted my own intentions regarding the person I intended to marry; I panicked and wavered, but each time the strength of my self-belief pulled me through. Around this time, when I said that I wanted to specialize in surgery, my father advised me against it, sincerely believing that I was not suited for the physical stress involved. He hauled me off to meet the Dean and Professor of Surgery. To my utter indignation Dr Shenoy, who I had worked with as an intern the previous year, proceeded to tell me why a woman wasn't cut out for the job. It was too arduous. 'You can be a fine physician,' he said. 'Or go for something like pathology, with fixed hours of work. More suitable for a woman.'

Later the same evening I wrote to Dr Bansod, seeking his advice. I want to be a surgeon. How should I proceed? I hesitated for a couple of days before dropping the envelope in the post-box. A few weeks later came his reply. 'You have the potential,' he wrote, and offered me sponsorship for training at the University of Liverpool in UK. 'I cannot advise you on your personal life. As for your career, please note that opportunities come once or twice in a lifetime. You must learn to seize them.'

I kept that letter folded between my hospital-wear saris—happy, sad and certain that my father would not let me go all by myself to another country. Months went by; my tenure in orthopaedics would be over in six weeks. Dr Gyanchand asked what I planned to do and I told him about the letter.

'You must show the letter to your father,' he said, chagrined. 'If he has any doubts, I will speak.'

How wrongly I foresaw my father's response. He was pleased. He did everything necessary to set me on course, travelling with me a number of times to Bangalore to apply for the passport and visa. Early November, my work-permit arrived from Liverpool and I was ready to go.

A few days before I left, I made a farewell visit to the hospital. Dr Gyanchand told me many things about England of the 1950s when he himself was a young aspirant. 'You've got to get the FRCS (Fellowship of the Royal College of Surgeons) from London,' he said. 'It's said to be the most difficult, but nothing is difficult.' He opened a wooden cabinet behind his desk and withdrew a thick green folder bulging with paper, along with a rectangular black box. The folder contained the notes he had made while preparing for the FRCS. Inside the box were six surgical instruments of the finest quality. 'Make good use of them.'

I mumbled my gratitude, said something about how undeserving I was of such kindness. 'If you can learn how to better use your faculties, you will finish your training and be back in three years,' he said, tersely. Cheeks aflame, I hurried out of his office. What he wanted from me was action, not obsequious gratitude.

In Bangalore, Dr Bansod invited me for a dinner with his family. A bit conceited perhaps, of my future prospects, I wore a slim-fit skirt in deep pink with a ruffled white blouse. (Whenever I make an attempt at sophistication, it races away ahead of me.) My efforts must have amused my host, I'm certain I saw a trace of hilarity in his eyes as I faltered into their sitting room on high heels. After dinner he sat me down for a talk. 'Take as long as you find it necessary to clear the FRCS. Work there for a while if you need to, but come back. There are no contractual obligations. But I expect you to work in India after training.' A grin broke over his face. 'Always remember that you represent our country. You will know, then, what to do in any situation.'

A knuckle-rap? I'm not sure but how I love the man for his words of caution. The three-and-a-half years I spent in England shaped my future in a very definite way.

6

England

Permanence and change are part of life. Change comes constantly and in many forms—as adjustment, a minor alteration, a complete transformation, or merely as a different perspective. It may come with great rapidity, or it may be so slow that you do not see it happen. Even so, change does not affect the permanence and certainty of immutable factors—the rising sun, the revolving earth, the laws of gravity and combustion; the fragile beauty of a flower, the constancy of love or faith; the marvel of survival in the face of hardship. It is best to accept both change and permanence in a sort of sisterhood with oneself.

Nervously stepping on a trundling escalator for the first time, I tripped and broke the strap of my slippers. It happened when the Air India flight from Bombay to London stopped in Paris for two hours and we disembarked while the plane was being refuelled. It was a cold night in November and I was a young woman in a fine silk sari, her moment of glory slightly diminished by the indignity of shuffling towards a seat and fixing the busted strap with a safety pin. London greeted me with its dismal grey skies and a freezing wind that wrapped itself around my ankles. The same afternoon I registered with the General Medical Council, and next day boarded the train to Liverpool, for six pounds-fifty.

Six hours later I got off at Lime Street Station which seemed to me like a dark hollow scooped out of the earth, built for lonely trains, and lonely travellers. The walls were black and people few.

The Royal Liverpool Hospital, better known as the Royal Infirmary, was a short walk up an incline called Pembroke Hill, which I could have walked, but for the cumbersome suitcase. I took a cab. The weathered, red-brick Victorian building, with its oak-and-glass-panelled entrance was like a grandmother of generous dimensions: affable and welcoming. The soft-featured, bulbous-nosed switch-board operator led me to my first-floor room. 'Any help you need, luv, give me a call,' said Tom. Thereafter I never left the hospital without stopping by at the switchboard for a chat whenever Tom was on duty. He became friend, counsellor and giver-of-directions.

Morning: shivering in my sari and cardigan I waited outside the Professor's office, clutching a packet of coffee and a miniature sandalwood elephant that I had brought for him. He came round his desk to greet me. He was courteous and precise: 'You will work as a casualty medical officer for six months and then in my surgical unit for a year. Time enough to prepare for part one of FRCS. Once that's out of the way, you can apply for a registrar's job. It gives you the surgical experience required to prepare for the finals.'

I was accustomed to being led by others; to having my life organized for me by others. I listened intently. 'Don't be in too much of a hurry to clear the exams,' he added. 'Prepare yourself well, for twelve to eighteen months perhaps, before appearing for part one.... Are you cold? You must get yourself some warm clothes, don't you think?'

Yes, I said, thinking how much he looked like John Kennedy. I handed over my gifts. 'Thank you. An elephant...! My daughter loves animals.' He pointed to a framed photograph of his family on his desk and then saw me off at the door.

The letter I wrote home that evening included a breathless paragraph about the professor.

I was one of the five casualty medical officers working with the pink, chubby Alfred Franklin, curly-haired Robin Mathews, rotundly handsome Dick Calver and the ultimate lady-killer Mike Evans. The nurse in charge of Casualty got me started next day and then it was work for eight hours, with a short break for lunch. We treated all emergencies: fractures, slipped discs, cardiac emergencies, insect bites, allergies, asthmatic attacks, the 'urgent' abdomens, suicide bids of every type, head injuries and febrile children; drug addicts, small-time criminals, malingerers and boozed up dock-workers. The rabble and the gentry came in a steady stream. There were dramatic, eye-popping moments of panic: barbiturate overdoses, slit wrists, comatose diabetics, gashed heads, road accidents. Then there were the really bizarre ones—like the young man who was brought in unconscious with a needle sticking out of his arm, or the tramp* with six months of body odour and in need of a few stitches on a cut thumb but more urgently a bath, a meal and a bed for the night. There were also the injuries inflicted by squabbling drunks or a soused spouse that kept us busy during the weekends. On my first Christmas night in Casualty, I played mediator between a quarrelling couple who had each clobbered the other and needed stitches on the head. As I worked on one, the other would come rushing in, spewing invectives, in an effort to complete the damage.

The job brought me quickly in contact with a variety of people: nurses, doctors, ambulance drivers, policemen, derelicts, old dears, and a few stuffed shirts. I could not have hoped for a better learning experience than those first few months at

---

*Tramps, I figured, were the equivalent of beggars—perhaps ever so slightly more genteel—with a great sense of the comic in everyday life. Only much later did I learn that they were the by-products of economic depression and unemployment.

the Royal Infirmary. There was newness as well as a feeling of familiarity about England, thanks to the long and persistent shadows of colonial occupation that stretch across Indian history. I did not miss home in any acute sense. When I felt like eating some good food, I would go across to one or the other of the Indian, Pakistani, Bangladeshi or Sri Lankan doctors' homes. They knew how to please fellow-sufferers, invariably, with chicken curry and rice. I walked the rain-sodden streets, trying with all my strength to resist the bullying winds. I went to the weekly party on Friday evenings. Sometimes, the Asian doctors arranged their own, with a Hindi film thrown in. The beer-swilling Fridays and the Indian parties (at which every one of us affected more Indianness than we could possibly be feeling, with silk saris and sherwanis) were disappointing. I soon gave them up. Some weekends I would visit a school friend who had been living in Luton after her marriage; or I dropped in on the Morrells, who were friends of Dr Bansod and lived a twenty-minute bus ride from the hospital. Many an English meal I have had with Eric and Laura Morrell while hearing them talk about the hardships of the war years. Eric was a retired baker. They were a couple of modest means and grateful to the National Health Service (for which I worked, like every doctor in the UK) which looked after their welfare.

At work and between shifts, there were wild and happy moments. To a generation of young doctors and nurses used to libertine enchantments, I was clearly a figure of curiosity and amusement. There was spluttering laughter when I declared earnestly that girls from India were always virgins before marriage. I listened to angst-filled accounts of Mike's girlfriends who thought I knew him well enough to gauge his affections. He married a few years later and went off to Wales. The lucky girl was not any of the nurses. A year later I realized that the clothes I bought for myself after carefully comparing prices were cheap and dowdy. Indians like myself, long used to the graces of middle-class restrictions of those times, spent sparingly.

Britain of the early seventies was kind to me in all sorts of ways. I fell under the spell of British charm, their composure and civility. What we in India convey with a nod, a smile, a raised eyebrow, a wave of the hand or tone, the Brits do with a 'Thank You'. 'Can I have a cup of tea, please, thanks.' 'Here you are, thank you.' 'Oh, thanks very much.' I once counted thirty-five thank-yous between a scrub-nurse and a surgeon during a surgery that lasted a little over an hour.

For me, life outside the hospital was comfortingly ordinary. My Asian compatriots (inside and outside the hospital) were few but varied: from India, Pakistan, Sri Lanka, Bangladesh, Nepal, Burma and from Uganda. Our similarities were more than the differences. Ramya arrived in Liverpool from Uganda around the same time as myself. She joined as a history student at a nearby college and we had run into each other at an Indian musical event. Her parents who owned a kindergarten school in Kampala had fled to England with their two sons and daughter to escape the brutalities of Idi Amin. The family set up a makeshift garment shop that sold cheap terylenes, gauzy curtains and imitation-lace in the basement of an unused parking lot. Along with dozens of others, these shops served low-income families, needy students and the unemployed. Ramya was one of the few friends I had outside the medical circle. She was quiet, sensible and determined. We got on very well together. Her great-grandfather had voyaged from Surat in Gujarat to Uganda as an indentured labourer in the 1850s. It was a three-year contract, but he stayed on to make a better life for himself and his family by setting up a grocery shop. The Indians had a good life in Uganda, said Ramya, until Idi Amin began to view them with suspicion and mistrust. She was an earnest, ambitious girl who finished her doctorate in African Studies and later became a professor at the University.

The British had wrapped themselves around the globe and called the shots for a few hundred years and now that greatness was a mere shadow. The Royal Infirmary was in the sunset years of its existence. Within a decade it would make way for an immense building of coarse grandeur, befitting the superfast progress and gadgetization of medicine. But when I was there, the city of Liverpool, along with its port and dockyards, was on the decline because of the downturn in the economy. Small family-owned shops were shutting down, making way for dazzling, many-storeyed department stores. The Beatles were already history, the pub where they sang every night on their way to fame was a pit stop for the few tourists who travelled to Liverpool. The small lanes and alleys were empty and desolate. Jobless dock-workers with flushed hypertensive cheeks and wheezy lungs frequented the Casualty department. An unhealthy diet, too much beer and too many cigarettes, coupled with stress caused by the financial debacle had ruined their health. We saw them all the time. Meanwhile, a determined stream of migrant job-seekers was flowing in. Career-conscious doctors like myself, students of law, history, language and art, porters and cleaners were climbing the social ladders. Edward Heath was prime minister and of more than passing interest because of his talent in music and his ultra-genteel mannerisms which provided excellent material for comedy shows. It was a time when racial hostility echoed through pockets of London and the trade unions called for reforms; history crunched its way forward.

In India, Sanjay Gandhi, the over-reaching son of the then prime minister, Indira Gandhi, was unclenching his fists. Letters I wrote and received were my link with family and friends. All by myself for the first time in my life, and learning, I was happy in the most complete way possible. There was no time for dark, dull thoughts.

7

Chirugia

When I wasn't on duty or window shopping, I was at the Harold Cohen Library which was a five-minute walk from my room and stacked ceiling-high with books. I went every day after work, carrying with me a small flask of coffee to see me through a few hours. In my room I wrote letters and read non-medical books. I envy myself those days of pure study, lonely walks and the pleasure of reading for free.

Lectures for surgical aspirants like myself were held on Wednesday and Saturday afternoons in a classroom across the quadrangle from the library. I was struck by the teachers' ability to simplify complex details, and the easy manner in which they related to students. Much of my free time was spent in study. A few months later when Mr Parry who taught Anatomy said, 'You're good. You can take the exam anytime,' I wasted no time in informing the professor. He eyed me with concern. 'You've been here less than six months. Give yourself at least that much longer,' was his advice.

I fidgeted. 'I'd like to try now, sir.'

'Well…if you've made up your mind…go ahead. I wish you luck. If you don't make it through the exams, don't take it too much to heart.'

I realize now that I had coerced him to (please) not stop me. When I passed, he invited me home to dinner along with the rest of his team. So it was a big deal.

The first six months in the Casualty department were over. My duties in the professor's surgical unit swung between wards, out-patients and the operating theatre. On Monday mornings, the professor held the Grand Rounds, when the entire team of two consultants, two registrars, the senior house officer (me), the house officer or intern, nurses and the physiotherapist participate. It was the high point of the week and came with its share of anxiety and expectations. Of the two consultants, Robert Sells, one of the earliest in the country to specialize in renal transplant, was in constant demand. He was voluble and flamboyant, with a remorseless sense of humour. The athlete's built, dark hair and sideburns were that of a dashing movie star. Never dull, he shared appallingly wicked jokes with the team during surgery. In the face of grim situations, he was unflustered, withdrawing into himself, softly swearing, not blaming anyone. When the operating list for the day was done he thanked his team, bowed to his scrub nurse, and changing into his everyday clothes breezed out.

Most days Sells sped off to other hospitals for emergency renal transplants. Sometimes he got stopped by the traffic police for disregarding traffic rules. Pointing to the ice-flask in the rear seat he would say: 'That's a kidney on its way to save a life. Want me to ditch the patient who's right now on the operating table, waiting for it?' They always let him go. Sells was a charmer, and forever the star.

The other surgeon, Albert Cusheri, was to Robert Sells as soup was to steak: portly, spectacled, soft-spoken and brilliant. In those fledgling years of hepatic surgery, he undertook precarious forays into the purple-red, rubbery, devilishly complex organ that perches below the right side of the rib cage. Its brooding quiet is deceptive. Made up of hexagonal cells, interconnecting tubules and a rich network of blood vessels, the liver is a busy place. It produces bile, digestive enzymes and other substances vital to health; it detoxifies harmful chemicals present in food. The liver is our in-house nutritionist working tirelessly to keep the body in fine fettle. A sick liver is bad news. It is a surgical nightmare to accidentally nick the liver with a scalpel, or to be confronted with one injured in an accident. Any delay in stopping the bleeding can result in fatal blood loss. Small rents can be sutured using a blunt 'liver needle' and sealed with gel-foam. In the 1970s, major surgery on the liver was hazardous.

By nature quiet and phlegmatic, Cusheri became animated when discussing the liver. He had been attempting to devise ways to defeat cancerous growths by transfusing anti-cancer drugs into the hepatic artery. Open surgery was the only way to do this until ultrasound scanning began and one could guide a cannula safely into place. The Cusheri operating lists went on forever. As a junior do-as-told assistant, I found it tiresome. Try as I might, the hand steadying the metal blade of retractor, which tugs at the open edges of the abdominal incision allowing the surgeon to operate with ease, would slacken. Cusheri would take the retractor from my hands. 'This way…'

The two registrars handled most aspects of patient care and surgery. One was a Jamaican I liked working with. It was the other, the senior registrar with his tricky Irish temper I avoided, in the beginning. If an emergency surgery had been scheduled for seven in the evening, his hectoring began at five: have you booked an anaesthetist? Is the blood ready? Have you checked his creatinine levels? The electrolytes? His temper went skyward several times a day. 'What you doing, luv? Kneading dough?' 'Pull up your socks, Miss, or try your hand at something else.' 'Like jump off the roof…' I once mumbled, trying to match his sarcasm.

'Not a bad idea,' he quipped. If everything went well, he gave me a hug. 'That's my darling…what on earth will I do if you go back to India?' One evening after a case, he leapt to his feet, declaring that he would teach us all an Irish folk dance. It all got a bit much and the theatre sister bundled us out.

The everyday tasks were mine to carry out, with help from the house officer: send the patient to theatre, draw blood, do the dressings, go to X-ray, call the anaesthetist, book a theatre, cancel the theatre, phone the boss, ask for the stretcher. Except for simple jobs like taking out a loosened toenail, draining a fluctuant abscess, removing warts or suturing a gash on the head, I assisted my seniors. Coordinated team-work shapes the outcome of surgery as much as individual skill.* Within the theatre complex of a busy hospital there are several operating theatres and as many surgical teams at work. The lists are pasted outside the theatre and the names of patients are crossed off when a case is done. Depending on the probable duration of each case, a list may have three cases; or ten.

The mornings start in good cheer. We exchange greetings, jokes and banter, happy to be ensconced within the double-doors of the operating complex, safe from the irritations that erupt in the wards and clinics. As the day wears on, problems begin to surface. And they keep coming.

'Who's clocked in this patient? Her asthma medications are not listed…'

'Sorry, dear, you'll have to let go off your dentures before I put you to sleep. You look just as good without them…'

'The suction's too feeble! What do you expect me to do, sister, carry a soup spoon in my pocket?'

'One gauze missing in the swab-count, doctor.'

'Your count's wrong. I know I've taken every one of them out…damn, here it is, hiding behind the uterus.'

Irritation grows, energy plummets, tempers unravel, at times beyond permissible levels. We argue, grumble, sulk and

---

*A surgeon once compared his team to the six horses which pull the sun's chariot: *Hraahm, Hreem, Hroom, Hroum, Hraim, Hraha*. The surgeon, anaesthetist, theatre sister, scrub-nurse, surgical assistant and the technician pulling the chariot, with the patient being the sun. A bunch of plumbers working together is perhaps more apt.

snap. The surgeon in charge becomes a target of displeasure. All we wish for is that the list be finished. We brush past each other in crumpled, bespattered theatre clothes, the masks leaving red weals on sweaty cheeks. When things go awry (as sometimes they do), the surgeon becomes a self-loathing wreck, frustrated and angry. Humour at times, comes to the rescue.

One of the senior gynaecologists, Mr T—— shared a story from his operating days with our team. That afternoon after a particularly difficult surgery on a uterine tumour, he was heading for the changing room, his surgical greens soaked through with blood. Mr Sells looked at him in mock dismay. 'Oh dear! Mr T—— Have you had a "period"?'

The moment would come when the last case on the list was crossed off. All I wished for was to lean back in a chair with a cup of tea, and *not* get up. But first there was the slow limp to the wards to check on the 'post-ops' and the critical patients.

Once in a while something big happened, dislodging the rhythm of work. An argument one forenoon between two surgeons on *who* was to operate on a patient ended in a tussle, with one shoving the other and he pinning his adversary (his boss) to the wall. It happened in a flash and then there was hell to pay, more so because one was an immigrant Indian doctor and the other a Brit. The Asian Doctors' Union got involved, and the media, with television channels interviewing the aggrieved individuals. There was another more tragic case of the wrong kidney being removed in a four-year-old girl resulting in her death. The surgeon was suspended from work; it became an ordeal for him to even step out of the house, for newspaper and television reporters pursued him everywhere. An accident like this would have finished an ordinary surgeon but this surgeon was not ordinary. His record of impeccable work, and petitions from scores of parents whose children had undergone major surgeries, spoke for him. The mother of the deceased child came out in his support. He was reinstated after seven months. I heard about the incident from the surgeon himself. It had been two years since the crisis blew over but the scar remained tender and hurtful.

A surgeon fixes the bodyworks when they get faulty. The *body* is the marvel, not the surgeon. The ability to ease pain and suffering and sometimes save a life sets a surgeon a quarter of a notch above other craftsmen who do similar work. Clean, plug, unplug, mend holes, remove decaying matter and debris; wash and clean and wash again. Most surgical ailments are caused by some form of mechanical obstruction that needs unblocking. About the process by which certain virulent bacteria release toxins which release gases that smell, you wouldn't want to know. Every hand that toils, gets soiled. If a surgeon did away with mask and gown and worked in the open beneath a tree or in an empty garage, if people saw and heard and *smelt* the reality of surgery, what then? Many of our near-and-dear would hesitate to eat with us and strangers would choose to walk on the opposite side of the road. Gachcha, gachcha.*

---

*In Sanskrit it means 'go away, go away,' a phrase made famous by Adi Shankara who used it against a low-caste chandala before he had a change of heart about the caste system.

8

Safaai Karmachari

I was five months into my surgical job and the Monday morning rounds were just over.

'A word with you,' said the professor, leading me to his office. 'You know the interviews for the registrar posts at the university are coming up?'

I did. There were twenty-one posts and lots of competition. The jobs promised the burden of academics, research and excellent work experience with noted surgeons.

'Why haven't you applied?'

I was twenty-four and heading towards a goal I had dreamed of for myself. I hadn't lost sight of it, but the momentum had flagged. I found myself disabled by dejection and self-doubt. It was all so difficult. What to do? Cut loose, make a neat U-turn and run back to the comforting folds of family and security? Change my course to something better suited to my wilting fervour? Get married quickly to my beau and sink into marital bliss? I could do all these things *and* be a surgeon, but that thought did not occur to me. What I do know is that had I given up on surgery, I would have lamented all my life.

I fought hard against my own faint-heartedness. Reading, walking, talking to myself, watching snowflakes drift through the deep windows of the Harold Cohen library as the steel-grey afternoon closed in and it was time for dinner. Quietly and stubbornly I survived the panic. But I wanted to run from anything that came with high expectations.

'I'd rather wait,' I told the professor, and tried to explain that I would prefer to be a low-profile surgeon in a less competitive district hospital than compete at the university level.

The blue eyes went cold steel. 'I don't have anything *easy* in mind. Go get the forms.'

With much misgiving, I applied. A deep sense of irritation at my own fickle nature, bouts of uncertainty and fears clouded the days that followed. Surgery is gendered territory, and comes with unspoken tensions for a woman, some imagined, others real. Achievements get noticed and failure is sniggered at. I had already come across male surgeons who were disgruntled by the 'foreign-body' (in more ways than one) in their midst. Sexual innuendos, unwanted physical contact, harassment and bullying, though rare, did happen. I managed to get past the unpleasantness, thanks to many factors which I will let be. I wanted something quiet and secure, but then—success is sweet, and I had been doing well all along. I struggled with my doubts.

The day of the interview arrived and there was some minor drama when I misread the location for the interview and went to the wrong place, about 11 kilometres away from where it was to be held. I rushed out of the wrong building, stumbled into a cab and explained as best as I could.

'Okey-doke,' the cabbie said, coolly and drove full speed. Halfway to our destination his cab stalled. Jumping out, he flagged another cab, shoved me in and wished me luck, and refused to take any money. I reached when all the candidates had finished and the actual selection process was on.

The selecting committee decided to relent and give me a chance. I was interviewed. Afterwards, while waiting for their decision, I got talking to the only other female candidate: Diedre Watson, a super-smart young woman from Guys Hospital, London. 'I want to be a cardio-thoracic surgeon,' she told me. Her hobby was to tinker with cars and bikes and second only to her love of surgery. We both made it and became friends. Diedre went on to realize her dream in the very competitive world of London hospitals where I met her years later as a cardio-thoracic consultant.

Next morning I was on my way to the professor's office when Sells summoned me. He led me to the annex where doctors met for tea. He was one of the seven or eight surgeons on the interview panel so obviously he wanted to convey his compliments—

'Disappointing performance,' he said, without a trace of humour in his voice. 'You got in because of your academic record. Why were you so dumb? Interviews give you a chance to speak, to tell the selectors that you are competent enough for the job. It's not for giving yes and no answers.' I could sense his anger. 'And let me ask, why are you so withdrawn at work? You must question, argue, disagree, confer. In theatre, ask for cases that you can do. *Aim* to be a surgeon, if that's what you want. Or you'll end up a shrinking violet all your life.'

And there I was, with a box of chocolates to distribute. I felt dreadful.

'It doesn't please me very much to tell you this, but you give me no choice.'

That was it. He opened the door and I stumbled out. After hating and avoiding him for days, I came to accept the truth of his words. Progress happens when you dare to overcome certain fixities of habit and conditioning. My learning was too methodical and passive. But I did not see myself as a shrinking violet. No!

I set to work on my inadequacies. Low-risk surgeries were there for the asking: appendix, hydrocele, hernia, vasectomy, the weekly 'lumps and bumps' list of day-cases surgeries. I took charge of patients and made my own decisions. On my call-duty days—which came three or four times a week—I handled the emergencies, at first operating with help from a senior and then doing them on my own. Every one of my seniors taught me surgical skills. Teaching a junior is not merely good practice but practical common sense. If a junior surgeon is good at her work, she is less likely to trouble her seniors at odd hours.

The work was incessant: 'acute abdomen' which is caused by gut that's blocked, twisted, ruptured or bleeding; burst ulcers, abdominal injuries, vascular, testicular, alementary, mammary, urinary and scores of other emergencies that came to hospital were routed usually through the Casualty department, where a few months ago I was doing the referral. Barring fractures which went to the bone specialist, a surgeon dealt with every surgical emergency. I learnt on the job. Years later when I met Sells, I reminded him of his words of reproach, which had been a turning point for me. He laughed. 'Now *I* feel embarrassed.'

In preparation for the final part of the FRCS, I made my pilgrimage to the Royal College of Surgeons in London, 'Royal' signifying the historic patronage by the British royalty (real or presumed). I spent several weeks in London visiting hospitals, attending lectures and clinical demonstrations that were being held for the Fellowship candidates. A room at the Indian YMCA on Fitzroy Square for three-pounds-fifty and the underground tube-transport were most affordable. The Royal College became my surgical sanctuary. Like a meditative praying mantis I gazed at the portraits of famed surgeons that hung on the walls, read volume after volume of the *Annals of the Royal College of Surgeons*, listened to exhilarating lectures by speakers whose work I knew of, observed specimens of a myriad diseases floating in glass bottles in the surgical pathology section and wandered goggle-eyed through the Hunterian Museum of Anatomy. History and knowledge streamed in the air. I became friends with several aspirants. We clicked photographs outside The Old Curiosity Shop and drank beer at the pub.

In my spare time, I immersed myself in the history of my

surgical forerunners. The ladder-high shelves of books at the library were my cache from which, bit by bit, I pieced together exciting events in the arc of medical progress.

9

Ancestor Worship

'Have a patient stand on a stool so as to get the fumes in his anus from the bark of chestnut, melon and old sandals on burning coals...'—Old Remedie for Piles. From a 14th-century manuscript*

The History of Medicine was not a core subject in medical colleges in India. It was taught to us at random intervals by a retired Major General from the Armed Forces Medical Corps. Statuesque, craggy-nosed, with sleek white eyebrows and attired in well-cut suits, Major General Bhatia was passionate about his subject. We heard out his lectures with vapid inattention, more fascinated by the pocketwatch that dangled on a gold chain from his vest than by his erudition, and thus deprived ourselves of history. I looked now to enlighten myself.

Caring is as old as human existence. The single most comforting sensation is that of touch—an inbuilt force of survival. The prehensile hand, the sensorial palm and the exquisitely designed digits enhance the emotional impact of touch. The crow furls its wings over the just-hatched fledgling;

---

*This directive was reproduced in a 19th-century advertisement by a doctor, with the postscript: 'Panic not! Be cured without sacrificing your sandals. Visit Dr Trim Tucker for a pain-free bottom.'

the mongrel licks away pain when her wilful pup snags a paw on a barbed wire; a mother-elephant soothes with her trunk. Humans are capable of helping any suffering being, even when not bound by love or loyalty. This ability to empathise sets us apart as a species. The other trait that is exclusively ours is hate. We'll stick with empathy.

Our cave-dwelling ancestors caressed their sick. Herbs, splints, smooth stones warmed by the sun, sharpened probes and oily emulsions of gum and resin were used to heal. If such common sense attempts did not help, there was witchcraft, prayer, mumbo-jumbo, acts of demonic music, dance, havans and sacrifice. Aesculapius in Greece and Dhanavantri in India were worshipped as gods of healing. At a temple to Aesculapius, the priest ministered to the sick, giving them advice purportedly spoken by the healing god, in his dreams. He thereby inscribed individual remedies on the walls of the temple. Dhanavantri was similarly deified, although some believe him to have been a worldly king with a sound knowledge of medicinal herbs. He died from snake-bite because there was no one with the skill to treat him.*

Greece and then Rome became the hub of early medical progress in the few hundred years that predate the Christian era. Hippocrates showed that by watching the patient move, speak, gesture and seat himself, by the fear in his eyes and the tremor of his fingers a physician could nail the malady. He noted everything that deviated from the normal, listened to the patient and thereafter predicted the disease and its course. At a time when dissection of the human body was unheard of, Hippocrates described the different ways in which a shoulder

---

*In parts of Kerala and Karnataka, there still exists a widespread belief in spirits and exorcism. In the month of Karkitakam (July-August) young boys of certain communities do the *Theyyam*, a ritual dance, to drive away the evil spirits which bring disease. Nowadays parents of these boys make sure that their sons participate only during weekends and holidays when the schools are closed.

or a hip could go out of joint in an injury. Certain methods of treatment which he described are still used, the best example being that of a dislocated hip. The Hippocratic method is to stand over the patient who lies on the ground and pull the limb upward, with a foot firmly pressing in the patient's groin for counter pressure. I have seen it done. The sound of the bone slipping back into place is very satisfying. This earliest of Greek masters is better known for laying down a charter of ethical medical conduct, based on which, doctors take the Hippocratic Oath. Galen, who came a few centuries later, was surgeon to the gladiators of Rome wounded in perilous sporting events. He described wounds as 'windows' through which the most grievous injuries could be understood. Galen learnt anatomy by dissecting apes. His premise of the to and fro motion of blood within the arteries was held as truth for over a millennium.

India was home to Sushruta, a remarkable surgeon who along with Charaka, a physician, lived about 2500 years ago. Sushruta's surgical expertise, swiftness and precision were hailed from the foothills of the Himalayas to the island kingdom of Lanka, from Dwaraka to Bodh Gaya. He refashioned noses, ears and breasts mutilated as punishment for adulterous women.* Cataract surgery was performed with a special curved needle and was one among the 108 surgical tools owned by Sushruta. He was also a famed urologist who removed egg-sized bladder stones in less than a hundred and twenty seconds, using the perineal method of extraction. What's more, he allowed potential customers to witness a surgery before giving consent. Only the bravest would agree to subject their private zones to a knife, beneath a tree, and without an anaesthetic.

Medical inquiry and knowledge thrived in ancient Egypt

*Soorpanaka ('she-of- the-sharp-claws') is said to have pleaded with Sushruta to make good her looks after the facial disfigurement she suffered as penalty for trying to seduce Rama, and then Lakshmana. Perhaps women like Soorpanaka reprised themselves with nails like claws.

and China. It flourished in the Arab world during the Middle Ages. The medical books written by Ibn Sena in 11th century CE were used in Italy, Vienna and several other parts of Europe for five hundred years. The dissection of human bodies became legal in the 17th century. In England, doctors were known to claim the bodies of beggars and the destitute, preserve them in formaldehyde and cut them open inch by inch. John Hunter and his brother William conspired with undertakers and grave-diggers to carry away corpses to use them for dissection and learning. Whispers were heard on the streets of London: a suspiciously large number of William Hunter's patients died at childbirth and the bodies were being ferried to the anatomy hall where his brother John waited to take charge of them. This was never proved, but an irrefutable case of poaching the dead is that of Charles Byrne the Giant, famous in London for his freakish looks, oversized bones and the sheer length of his body.* John Hunter had a passion for collecting the skeletons of animals and abnormally structured humans and had begged the Giant to bequeath his skeleton to the collection. A furious Byrne refused, and made a record of his desire to be protected from such brazen doctors. He wished to be buried after death. Hunter bribed the undertakers a royal sum of 500 pounds sterling in exchange for all seven feet and seven inches of the Giant. The coffin filled with rocks and stones was buried with due ceremony. The remarkable skeleton of Charles Byrne greets visitors at the entrance to the Hunterian Museum at the Royal College of Surgeons in London. Byrne seems to be taking it in good humour.

The real kinship of surgeons is with barbers who preceded us in the craft of *chirugia*. Kitted with scissors, blades, probes

---

*He suffered from a condition called acromegaly or gigantism, caused by a serious disruption of hormones produced by the button-sized pituitary gland fastened to the base of the brain. Gigantism equals the opposite of longevity, so Charles Byrne was fortunate to live till his thirties.

and tweezers, using salves, astringent lotions, soapy water, a mirror and towel, the barbers snipped off the ugly wart or the unbecoming mole, cut into painful phlegmons releasing odorous pus, evicted ticks feeding inside an ear or nose, picked out a thorn embedded in the finger or grit out of the eye. A disfiguring lump, a painful abscess, a stiff neck? Seek out the barber's shop right there on the street and allow his skilled hands to do the job. The medical community was jealous: these coarse men with blades and clippers are stealing our patients! The cannier among them snatched the snip-and-cut skills of barbers and made it their own, and they were the surgeons.

The surgeons who had inherited their skills from barbers were frowned upon by the physicians. The aggressive nature of surgery, the physicians felt, was not becoming. Surgery could not be the equal of their own more knowledgeable status and therefore surgeons were disallowed medical membership. This rivalry went on for years before the surgeons decided to break away. Thus, was formed the Royal College of Surgeons in 1800. The British surgeons still insist on being addressed as a Mister, Missus or Miss but never Doctor, thus emphasizing their exclusive legacy.

Europe was the hub of medical progress from 17th century CE. Two hundred years later, across the Atlantic, Northern America began to assert itself with refreshing audacity and sharp thinking in contrast to the punctilious plodding of their European kin.

It was 1809. Dr Ephraim McDowell, working in a small town in Kentucky, agreed to remove an ovarian tumour in a woman while she lay on her kitchen table reading from the Bible. There was no anaesthesia, if you overlooked the solace provided by the Holy Book, and the kindlier one of a tot of brandy. McDowell readied his instruments, laid out the ligatures, flexed and extended his fingers and felt the lady's pulse. The villagers gathered outside. They came prepared to settle scores if he failed.

McDowell reached for the knife that he had just sharpened on the grinding stone and made a sure, sharp, four-inch incision from the umbilicus downward, choosing the midline where the bleeding would be minimal. Almost immediately he sighted the transparent glistening peritoneum that covers the abdominal organs. Pinching up this thin layer between two fingers of his left hand, he cut through it and entered the cavity in which, partially screened by loops of bowel, gleamed the melon-smooth tumour, twice the size of a newborn head. With a measured sweep of the fingers, he freed it from the slithering coils of gut until he reached the stalk, with the purple, engorged blood vessels that fed the tumour. Without a moment's hesitation he pushed his index finger firmly around the pulsing vessels, tied them with a length of strong linen that his wife used to mend clothes and then cut through to detach the melon. He sewed up the belly with a single stitch.

'The fruit of my labour, gentlemen!' he cried, holding aloft the tumour in his bloodied hands in full view of the faithless villagers. Then he washed his hands and felt the lady's pulse. 'You can close the Holy Book for now, have another swig of brandy and get some sleep,' he said to the brave woman.

The surgery was over in two minutes. The patient survived. McDowell, who deserves to be a posthumous fellow of every prestigious surgical institution, had the classic requisites of a good surgeon: skill, speed, courage (some might call it audacity) and perfect judgement.

Theodore Billroth in Vienna, Austria, was the first surgeon to venture into the upper portion of the abdomen, excise a portion of the stomach for a cancerous growth and restore gut continuity by sewing the cut ends of bowel together. For years, while scrubbing for surgery I would invoke Billroth whose technique for excising portions of the gut laid the foundation for gastro-intestinal surgery. The main drawback to such difficult and lengthy procedures was the lack of an effective agent—other than opium or alcohol—to deaden pain. In the late 19th century, it became known that distilling sulfuric acid (vitriol) with alcohol produced 'sweet vitriol' or ether. It gave a pleasant high when inhaled and its use as a recreational drug was all the rage.* Nitrous oxide or Laughing Gas made its debut as an anaesthetic agent in the US and chloroform in Edinburgh and like ether, they were highly sought after at parties. Queen Victoria agreed to take chloroform during the birth of her second son, Leopold. In her Majesty's own words, the experience was 'soothing, quieting and delightful beyond measure'.

The impact of anaesthesia was dramatic. It became the most important aide to surgery, changing the very personality of its practitioners forever. Listen to medical man in Bernard Shaw's *A Doctor's Dilemma*:

> In my early days, you made your man drunk; and the porters and students held him down; and you had to set your teeth and finish the job fast. Nowadays you work at your ease; and the pain doesn't come until afterwards, when you've taken your cheque and rolled up your bag and left the house. I tell you, chloroform has done a lot of mischief. It's enabled every fool to be a surgeon.

Nevertheless, surgeons could now dare to venture anywhere in the body. Anaesthesia provided the time to handle tissues gently and respect anatomical detail. Surgery became precise, safe and attractive; surgeons, bold and theatrical. Even now, we are unwilling to shake off the aura, unable to resist being photographed with a surgical mask dangling over the chin. In the early decades of the 20th century, medical schools of Europe had operating rooms (fittingly referred to as theatres)

*I did not have this delicate piece of information when I dripped ether over gauzed masks to anaesthetize patients with fractures. The Almighty-caretaker-of-surgeons was clear about what I should know.

with tiered seats around the central stage—the operating table—where surgeries were performed before an audience. The surgeon, dressed in his street clothes decorated with blood stains, would excise an offending piece of tissue and hold it up; the rapt audience of doctors and students would applaud. Showmanship was part of being a surgeon. Ambroise Pare, surgeon to four kings of France, subverted such pomposity by reminding surgeons that they only dressed wounds. The Almighty healed.

Ignaz Semmelweis who beseeched surgeons to wash their hands before any operation or delivery paid for his discovery with the loss of his professional status, his sanity and eventually his life, because no one believed the truth of it. He did not know then that it was the bacteria (streptococcus pyogenes) that were being carried from the cadavers to the young women in labour.* A decade later, the germ theory became known when Louis Pasteur, a chemist, discovered the use of vaccines as an effective barricade against deadly diseases.

Joseph Lister, the Professor of Surgery in Glasgow, had read about microbes that caused infections. It was at the time common practice for wounds to be left to 'suppurate', in other words to let the pus pour out while nature took its course. Lister had found that certain chemicals like carbolic acid (used in the cleaning of sewers) was effective against microbes. The opportunity to try it on patients presented itself in 1865, in the form of a young boy whose leg was severely crushed under a moving cart. The bones were splintered, the muscles and skin were torn and bleeding profusely. After an emergency surgery, Lister left the wound open, without suturing the skin, because of the likelihood of infection that would be even more dangerous if trapped beneath sutured skin. He soaked a piece of lint in carbolic acid and placed it over the open wound, and

*See Chapter 21 for Ignaz Semmelweis's story in detail.

changed the dressing every day. To his surprise, there was no infection and six weeks later, the boy hobbled out of hospital.*

Lister introduced the washing of hands before surgery and the cleaning of surgical instruments with carbolic acid. In 1867, he published the result of his work in *The Lancet*. Sterile surgical technique became the norm and brought an end to the grandeur of blood-splattered surgical gowns and unsterile instruments.

It was William Stewart Halsted, a surgeon at John Hopkins in the US, who introduced the use of gloves. It is best described by him:

> In the winter of 1889 and 1890—I cannot recall the month—the nurse in charge of my operating room complained that the solution of mercuric chloride produced a dermatitis of her arms and hands. As she was an unusually efficient woman, I gave the matter my consideration and one day in New York requested the Goodyear Rubber Company to make, as an experiment, two pair of thin rubber gloves with gauntlets. On trial these proved to be so satisfactory that additional gloves were ordered.

This wonderfully thoughtful gift of gloves sealed a romance. Halsted married the nurse, Caroline Hampton. And surgeons have worked with washed and gloved hands ever since.

The removal of an appendix, like a tonsillectomy or hernia repair, ranks low in status among surgeries. It is one of those first bread-and-butter procedures to be mastered by an apprentice. Perfection in what may seem like simple surgeries is like perfecting your daal and rice, or a cup of tea, but there is more to it than technical skill. A seemingly useless organ, the appendix was the cause for high drama when it struck two famed

---

*Surgeons operating on injured soldiers during wars have found this method to be valuable. The technique is still used in severely contaminated and crushed wounds, in order to save life and limb.

personalities. After the death of Queen Victoria and a few days before his coronation in 1902, Prince Edward VII fell ill with acute appendicitis. The treatment was—and is—immediate surgery. Anaesthesia was in its adolescence and antibiotics that fight wound infection were unknown. The surgeons hesitated, fearing complications that could prove fatal. When the prince showed no signs of improvement, they sought the advice of Lister, the foremost surgeon of the time. He advised them to go ahead with surgery, with proper attention to scrupulous antisepsis. The operation was a success and the coronation took place, with solemn splendour, the still-bandaged belly of the king draped in layers of royal apparel.

Our own Mohandas Karamchand Gandhi came down with appendicitis in 1924. At that time he was serving a six-year sentence at Yeravada Jail in Pune. Surgeons saw, and they dithered. Gandhi was fragile, fifty plus and fussy about food. Surgery was the treatment of choice. But was it not better to wait and watch? This second-best line of treatment where the surgeon uses conservative methods first is called the 'masterly inactivity' of withholding surgery. Gandhi's condition worsened and surgery became the only option. Colonel Maddock at Sassoon Hospital of Pune agreed to operate. It was a night of a fierce thunderstorm and during the surgery, just as the angry, swollen appendix burst at its tip, discharging pus into the abdominal cavity, the electric light fused and darkness closed in over the operation site. Maddock completed the procedure by the light of a hurricane lamp. The nation woke next morning to the smiling face of their beloved leader on the front pages of the newspapers. A national tragedy had been averted. A failure would have been a catastrophe. Gandhiji's prison term was cut short after the illness and he was discharged from prison soon after.

The decision to operate was sound judgement in both cases. I wonder how the two men would have reacted to the fact that their illness was largely the result of a bad diet with low-fibre content. Gandhiji ate a narrow range of natural but low-residue foods (and did not drink enough fluids); Prince Edward was a hearty eater and drinker at a time when the British diet had little roughage. Hardened* faecal matter would have obstructed the appendix in both men, encouraged the proliferation of harmful bacteria and caused infection.

*The technical term is 'inspissated' and is somehow more apt.

10

Plumbing Away...

I do not remember much about the final exams, except that it was a calm and laidback affair which put most of us at ease. On being questioned about thyroid surgery I explained at length, quoting the thyroid specialist, Hilary Wade, whose work I had read. I remember the moment when my name was called out among the successful candidates and finding out that the examiner who asked me about the thyroid was none other than Hilary Wade. I remember being congratulated by the examiners for clearing the exams at a young age.

On the train back to Liverpool, I wrote letters to convey the news home. An international call booked through a telephone operator was a luxury reserved for more urgent matters.

*

A month later I got married to the young man I had decided to marry in Liverpool. He was a year senior to me in medical college and had come to England a year before me. Those were wonderful, wonderful days, in spite of the fact that my own family was unhappy about it. Life was good in every way possible. Personal happiness enhanced my efficiency at work. There is a moment in the learning of every skill when it no longer feels like something that is difficult to master but more like music, or a lightness of step which becomes a part of you. I steadily improved my surgical skills. When the eighteen months as registrar were nearing completion, I got a much sought-after surgical job at the 1500-bed Walton Hospital. One of the four registrars who was to be one of my colleagues greeted me with: 'You'll see. It is so busy here, it's difficult to make time for the loo.'

I worked for two senior consultants. One was boyish, sweet and somewhat volatile. He treated me like a friend. The only thing that riled him was shoddiness at work. His colleague, with his swarthy skin, black-rimmed spectacles and the I-know-exactly-what-I'm-doing kind of smile looked a lot like Henry Kissinger. But unlike Kissinger, this man was genuine and fearless in the gravest of situations; and a tough person to work for. He had special interest in vascular surgery whereby diseased or injured segments of blood vessels are excised and grafts used to bridge continuity. It amazed me how this man who advised his patients against smoking because nicotine damaged the blood vessels was himself never without a cigarette (for longer than absolutely necessary). When the operating lists were decided on—the evening before—I would try to settle for cases that were predictable and safe. He realized what I was up to and insisted on giving me challenges.

'Show me you can do it,' he would say cheerfully. 'I'm in the other theatre, you can always call for help.'

Once, opening a patient with cancer stomach, I found that the growth had extended well beyond its walls, tethering it to loops of the small bowel, the gall bladder and the uterus. 'An open-and-shut case, I'm afraid,' I said to the anaesthetist and asked him to convey it to the boss in the next room. Kissinger strode in to have a look. 'Umm...have you checked the liver for secondary deposits? It's clear? Oh good, then you must just get on with it, you know. Yes, the stomach, the uterus and those bits of gut adhering to the uterus...the omentum...everything.

Out! Don't leave behind any lymph nodes, either, mind you.' I tried to explain that it was too much for me. 'I'm sending you another assistant,' he said, grinning as he walked away. It was the first case on my list. Five and a half hours later I closed the belly. My clothes were soaked through. I was mercifully let off, for a bath and some food and the other cases on my list were postponed.

There is much to learn by observing others. Mercurial temper, indecision, arrogance and incompetence are the negative qualities I learned to avoid. My own negative qualities—impatience, laziness, timidity and the tendency to be too quickly judgmental—threatened to trip me up as dangerously as the first escalator I stepped on in Paris.

A few choice examples of the oddities among the surgeons are too good to miss. There was the courteous and courtly Lord Burgess—born into a distinguished family of peers. When I met him, he was retired and well past his prime but continued to attend hospital and operate. It was a voluntary goodwill gesture which no one dared question. It had as much to do with his likeable nature as with his peerage. Burgess displayed a mild contempt for the new and the unfamiliar—be it an instrument, a gadget or a technique—and dismissed all things new as needless extravagance or 'jiggery-pokery'. He charmed patients with his graciousness and disarmed the younger, more versatile surgeons with equal felicity. I once assisted this grand old man for a prostate surgery. In the midst of a rather bloody procedure, he dropped his thickly rimmed black spectacles into the wound leading horrified gasps from scrub-nurse, anaesthetist and assistant. But Burgess simply fished out the spectacles from the wound. 'Clean it with a wet gauze, will you?' he said to one of the nurse-aides. He had them back on in seconds and continued with the surgery.

One of the older matrons in the hospital told me about Mr E——, a gynaecologist, who liked to operate without gloves.

This was a century after Semmelweiss and Lister and several decades after the wearing of gloves became a part of surgical discipline. Mr E—— held the belief that bare hands were better for the fine art of surgery and did away with gloves. He even did the internal examination of women with bare hands. The matron who told me about him had been a student in his time. He was apparently very popular with his patients but his colleagues were outraged. It sorted itself out eventually when he retired and not one of his juniors showed the inclination for bare-handed surgery.

I knew Dr C—— as a House Officer. He was tall and studious-looking, with a high-school slenderness to his body and a pubescent pinkness to his cheeks, a small head of tight black curls and ultra-magnified glasses. Walking into the wards in the morning, I always saw young C—— bent over a patient like a sheathed white tube of disaster. I never saw anyone with such a violent pair of hands. C—— did not insert a needle, he plunged it; he did not open a sterile packet of sutures, he tore into it; he thrust tubes with fierceness into unsuspecting patients. One can only admire the stoic calm of those men and women who took the insult. Simple, everyday procedures like introducing a urinary catheter or setting up an intravenous line finished with blood-splattered sheets, a pale, sweaty patient slumped and a fretful young nurse biting back her fears. I tried talking to C—— about it but he either did not see my point, or was clever enough to divert the conversation towards, of all things, religion. He was pursuing the study of some grim cult of Christianity and vehemently believed that terrible punishments are in store for sinners. I have no idea what happened to Dr C——.

One of the best surgeons I worked with was Averil Mansfield, who showed that a woman could not only be among the best, she could be *the* best. She was not merely a very skilled surgeon in the technical sense, her surgical judgement was unerringly perfect, her demeanour firm but modest. I loved working with this fine woman. Presence of mind—that's what she taught me. I am certain that it improved my surgical abilities. (Shamefully I admit, it did nothing for the absence of mind which overtakes me in certain other departments.) Averil Mansfield went on to head surgery at a leading hospital in London where about a decade later, I met her, shortly before her retirement. She had aged, but was as modest and friendly as ever.

Gender bias does exist but it is not unbreachable. Racism, which is made much of, is not anything as bad for Indians as the caste and class divide that we have in our own backyard. Professionally, I did not face racism in Britain. I was pulled up for mistakes and rewarded when I performed well. Petty instances did surface occasionally. It happened to me late on a Sunday evening when I was called to Casualty to see a patient with a chest injury. The man had broken four ribs; a fragment had punctured the lung causing air to leak out of it. His breathing distress was obvious. Having checked him and the X-rays, I explained that a tube would be inserted into the chest cavity to drain out the leaking air, allowing the lungs to expand and normal breathing to be restored. When the nurse asked the patient to sign the consent form, he said, 'No foreign doctor for me, thanks. I want one of *our* doctors.' The nurse tried to reassure him but he did not budge. '*She's* going to stick tubes into me chest? Nope.'

I had heard good things about myself, professionally, and was unprepared for this refusal by a patient, that too, a man gasping for breath. 'That's fine by me,' I snapped. 'Sister, I'm off. There's plenty to do in the wards.' I went to my room to sulk; the matron called, and then the anaesthetist called. No surgeon other than me was on duty until Monday morning. 'Not my fault,' I said, still angry. The administrative staff who vanished from the precincts after duty hours hurried back to resolve the crisis. Eventually, my phone rang. The patient had made a formal apology, so would I please return to work? I was relieved; I did not really want his condition to worsen.

*

It was time to think of going back home. Returning to India after living in another country isn't easy. For us, there were innumerable concerns, mostly trivial, but they did not appear so at that time. It created a sense of un-belonging and perplexity. I wrote to friends and relatives; a diary I kept during those years was like writing letters to myself, a sort of self-questioning about my intentions. Medical school, internship and post-graduate studies had taken nine years of my life. I had two degrees to my name and anxieties caused by high expectations. I had no doubt about wanting to work in India but what would it be like? Within the privileged class to which I belong, we do not hold ourselves responsible for the miseries of those beyond our territory. We are brought up to be kind to our domestic help and sympathetic to the workers who till our paddy fields and preserve our coffee plantations so that we may live in comfort, get educated and be assured of continued wealth and comfort. Life on other side of the chasm remains an unpleasant blur.

I had no interest in politics. That my father had joined the freedom struggle and devoted his entire life to politics was one of the verities with which I lived. At times he told us about his years in prison, the hardships as well as the inspiring moments he spent in the company of some of our foremost leaders. All of it was inspiring but somehow far removed from the immediate problems that concerned me.

I had begun to question my own attitude and prejudices. My husband was keen on higher training in the US; and during my term at Walton hospital in Liverpool, he worked in Boston and then in San Antonio, Texas. Towards the end of this final tenure, we found ourselves pulled in an altogether different direction. I had decided to work at our medical college hospital in Bangalore and was in the process of completing the paperwork required, when a tattered blue aerogramme reached me. It was a letter from a friend, Sister Ancilla, urging us to work at Nazareth Hospital in Bihar, which was desperately in need of doctors.

I remember holding that letter in my hand; wondering. *Bihar*? Surely not Bihar? By the end of the day I was thinking, why *not* Bihar?

Friendships are made and unmade; strangers provoked; colleagues flattered, pleased and displeased through epistles. Letters, memos, scribbles, email and SMS are the silent messengers of thought. It is fascinating to think that the earliest missives were scratched with the fingernail on mud, with a sharp stone on a tree-bark, with blood on a rock, perhaps. Life-altering decisions happen because of the communicated word. For me, the written word is more pleasing than a phone call and sometimes works almost as well as a face-to-face talk. (As for Skype and web conferences, I worked hard to stay clear of them until the Coronavirus pandemic made it a necessity.)

Sister Ancilla and I were friends from our college days. She was the only one who could get me out of bed very early in the morning and to her room with the promise of coffee brewed using a thumb-sized electric coil. Although a decade older to the rest of us in college, Ancilla was game for all things fun, including, once a rum-and-cigarette session in the girls' hostel. But it was the early morning coffee that did it. Terms and conditions included being in her room at 6 a.m. sharp for an hour of study. Now she was tempting my husband and me with the allure of working in a part of our country that was north and east of everything I knew…

11

The National Health Service

'Look to your health; and if you have it praise God, and value it next to a good conscience; for health is the second blessing we mortals are capable of.'—Izaac Walton

After returning to India, I did go back to England a few times over the years to update skills and increase my ability to handle a broad range of surgery. They were shorter stints lasting six to eighteen months at a time. I must give a brief overview of the health service in Britain, for it is a system that has served the country very well.

In the century preceding the World Wars, doctors in Britain were self-employed or taken on hire by industries and business houses. In rural towns and villages, the doctor trudged miles or rode on horseback to reach his patients, carrying his battle weapons and medicines stuffed in a bag.* For many leading physicians and surgeons, London was the place to be in. The most fashionable among them chose Harley Street, an upper-

*As a high-school girl I used to shed tears over the romance of the medical world in novels. I read those touching, at times over-sentimental, works of A.J. Cronin; Richard Gordon's madly aberrant fables of doctors' lives; and the veterinary tales of James Herriot, which are as much about the animals he treated as they are about the people who own them. The element of truth was never far from these works.

class housing locality in Marylebone. In 1860 there were twenty doctors in the area; at the turn of the century 200 physicians worked in these hallowed clinics. Of the well-known residents of Harley Street were the landscape artist J.W. Turner, the handsome and gifted psychoanalyst Masud Khan from Lahore, Charles Wilson the personal physician to Churchill, and Lionel Logue the Australian speech therapist who helped King George VI overcome his stammer. Harley Street now boasts of 3000 medical professionals. They treat the rich and famous for every sort of disorder, from chipped nails and ankles aching from high heels to insomnia, the food and bodyweight dilemma, neuroses and other more genuine illnesses. Nationality and colour no bar, the only requirement is a kingly income.

By 1945, a war-ravaged Britain found itself faced with grave concerns of economy. The Labour government wanted to make socially relevant changes in welfare and education. The economist William Beveridge proposed a plan for a nationalized welfare system in which every earning citizen would pay a regular sum as contribution towards medical insurance. Medical care would be universal. National insurance is thus totally unlike private insurance schemes which offer services depending on the premium paid. Beveridge believed in social welfare which ensured a minimum standard of living, *below which no one should be allowed to fall.* A healthy workforce was essential if the country was to recover. A wise man had spoken and the government listened. The details of the National Health Service (NHS) were worked out by the health ministry headed by Aneurin Bevan and the NHS Act was passed by the Parliament in 1948. The doctors treating the 55 million citizens of the country were directly employed by the government. The Labour Party was in power when NHS was introduced. Nevertheless, subsequent governments have seen its merits and have ensured its sustainability and quality.

Within the NHS, two streams of medical services work

in tandem. The general practitioner (GP) or family physician provides first-step care. General Practitioners work in groups of two to four. If a doctor goes on leave, she arranges a temporary replacement (a locum) to do her job, be it for weeks, months or a few hours. Young doctors in hospital practice who wish to earn extra money fill these short-term vacancies. The doctor-patient relationship built over the years is crucial to the quality of care and early detection of disease. Hospital-based doctors treat those who need more advanced treatment or surgery, admit and do surgeries as necessary.

The career possibilities in the NHS are good and rest entirely on competence. Once a doctor reaches the level of a senior registrar, she can apply for the permanent post of a consultant anywhere in the country. It becomes possible for the family to settle down and enables the doctor to work closely with the local community, thus enhancing one's professional and personal life. Part-time work is permitted to women, which is essential for many during the early years of child-bearing. Private practice is restricted, tightly regulated and open only to consultants. It is of no advantage whatsoever to a patient, except for the exclusivity, and an early appointment. For those who do not have to worry about high costs, it might be more convenient, but certainly only for uncomplicated cases. The success of the NHS led to its duplication in the commonwealth nations of Australia, New Zealand and Canada.

The NHS is an excellent social welfare system which, at times, is taken undue advantage of. Patients are quick to dial the medical emergency service to summon an ambulance (free) for trivial complaints; the service is misused by malingerers, hypochondriacs, bibulous knockabouts or the occasional family trying to shrug off an ageing parent by depositing her/him at the hospital.

To add to this, the rising costs of drugs, administrative expenditure and the wastage of disposable items in hospitals have not been curtailed. Misuse and wastage within the NHS have caused a steady leakage of resources, bringing it under the attack of disgruntled patients and those who believe in privatized medicine. This includes a lobby of medical professionals who have been demanding privatization of health. In spite of these drawbacks, NHS—if restructured and more tightly controlled—is a marvellous system for providing universal health care.

12

Why Not Bihar?

Hospitals in Europe began as hospices where the terminally ill and the dying sought relief. Succour for the anguished was integral to the life of Jesus Christ. In India, Sri Ramakrishna and Swami Vivekananda pragmatized the virtue of karma and pressed monks into the service of fellow-men. Shelters, ashrams and dharamsalas aided by generous benefactors reached out to the destitute and sick. Western missionaries (who followed the colonizers) trudged through jungles, tribal belts, hill-districts and barren stretches, combining evangelization with medical care, and later, education. They set up hospitals in difficult situations, well before the government awakened to its importance. In Islam, zakat is a concept by which a good Muslim is expected to give 2 per cent of his or her personal wealth to those in need. This is a way of implementing social welfare through the medium of faith. I saw it in action at two government-aided hospitals in Karachi where voluntary donations make it possible to provide quality care in serious illnesses like cancer and renal failure. Outside one of the largest government hospitals were makeshift shelters for the relatives of patients who came from great distances and who sometimes stayed for months. They were fed and clothed by the citizens of the neighbourhood.

Karuna. Caritas. Zakat. They are all an expression of

the primal and intuitive force of caring. Religious and other organized units tap into this force which already exists in us. Speaking for myself, I have never been religiously inclined. Perplexed by the tenets and contradictions that come with every religion, I have tried to keep a safe distance from matters holy. I live with my impiety, in closeness with religion. My own community of Kodavas are ancestor-worshippers who came in contact with Hinduism about 300 years ago; my husband was a brahmin but not rigid in any way; I studied in convent schools for several years, did my medical training at the only Catholic medical college in India and went on to work in three mission hospitals—two Christian and one Hindu. One out of these three was the finest in my medical experience and another, the worst.

When he returned home from England, our families welcomed us with affection. It was not easy for anyone—it never is—to meet tradition halfway. The distress caused by a 'love marriage' is due to needless and wrongly perceived notions of family honour. My dream for future generations is a world where inter-caste, inter-religion and inter-racial marriages are accepted with as much ease as a Punjabi eating idlis or a Saraswat brahmin reaching for mutton biryani. When members of one family embrace more than one faith, the customs, food habits, and the sometimes suffocating grip of tradition become less relevant. Health-wise too, it bodes well: there will be a dramatic decrease in inherited diseases.

Having visited our homes in the south, we went to Bihar. Mokama is a rural town 90 kilometres south of Patna. It is best known as the home of dacoity in and outside the state; it is also where Jim Corbett worked as a contractor supplying coal to the railways. It was here that one evening while having a bath he found himself in the company of a cobra. Trying to contort himself into a position of safety he knocked down the oil lamp and managed a narrow escape. Mokama is also where in the late 1940s, four American nuns set up a dispensary on an arid maidan half a kilometre from the railway junction. Local transport consisted of two hand-held push-carts. By the end of the 1970s, when we were there, the push-carts had made way for half a dozen cycle-rickshaws.

The nuns belonged to the holy order of the Sisters of Charity of Nazareth, with its Mother House in Kentucky and in the early years, many of the doctors and nurses were American. In thirty years, they had a hospital of 150 beds with a nursing school and trained staff. Very early in the mornings patients would arrive at the outpatient department where six doctors (sharing two cubicles) would see them. By 8 a.m. patients would press forward at the entrance, by 10 a.m. they would be heaving, lunging and shoving in the true and only fashion of our countrymen. We managed. Four of the younger doctors, including me, also did night and weekend shifts. Mid-morning, I would wait longingly for the tea that arrived from the hospital canteen; a few hours later I would peel off my white coat, duck low and make a quick escape to our living quarters upstairs.

The nuns took good care of us. The hospital kitchen supplied freshly baked bread. A chapel and a Jesuit monastery abutting the hospital housed a priest and a handful of seminarians. Wheat, rice and pulses were grown on a few acres of land around the monastery. This absurdly magical part of our country provided both of us—my husband and I—with lasting gifts of knowledge and experience.

The operating theatre was under the serene and strict eye of Ms Bernadette and her team of nine tribal girls. Bernadette had been picked by an American surgeon years earlier when, as a girl of seventeen, she had come in search of a job. She was small and slight with tranquil eyes that saw thousands of grisly cases and many surgeons—quirky, brilliant and mediocre—over the thirty-eight years she worked there. Her zone of discipline included the operating theatre and also the sterilization and packing units. Bales of gauze and cotton were cut and fashioned into wound dressings, glass syringes in individual wrappings were autoclaved and labelled, the theatre cleaned as per the strict rules of asepsis. Bernadette or one of her team took turns to assist at operations. The system was tuned to an effective level of efficiency because of which we could handle serious emergencies within twenty minutes of their being brought to the hospital.

Mokama is an unpredictable world of violence and peace, of Bhumihars and bonded labour, child brides, courteous men with guns strapped at the waist, the trusting and the untrustful. I was young and keen to show off my skills. However, a few weeks into my job, I felt like a hack with two left hands. No one had taught me how to deal with gunshot wounds that respect no rules and always chance it at night; gas gangrene of the lower limb in full-term pregnancy; fractured femurs in ladies with chalk-brittle bones; gallstones, kidney stones, kilo-weight spleens, torn livers, gaping chests; and infants with tetanus and diphtheria. A few good textbooks were my only teachers. My anaesthetist, a nurse who had been informally trained, would smile encouragingly. 'Just get on with it,' is what her smile said. For years Bihar had been entrenched in poverty, feudal oppression and everyday spurts of violent crime. Combined with extremes of weather, corruption and an indifferent government, the average Bihari was reduced to hopeless timidity. Health was indeed a luxury: malaria, kalaazar, worm infestations, parasitic diseases, cholera, diphtheria and leprosy presented in the most severe forms. The hospital itself, being inexpensive and well-maintained, attracted patients from outlying villages and the towns of Beguserai, Batinda, Barauni and Arrah. Cleanliness aids recovery and who better than a bunch of dedicated nuns to create a pattern for a simple, clean and orderly environment? They achieved it through years of perseverance in the face of danger and hardship that would have scared away many a daring swashbuckler. We worked with the confidence of a team aware of our ability and limitations.

Looking back at the young surgeon I was, I see the purposefulness, and the arrogance. I became used to the working conditions in Bihar that were vastly different to those in Britain and often had to be handled in a special way. Undernourished patients, the local customs, outdated equipment, unbelievably frequent power cuts and a shortage of vital supplies influenced the outcome of surgery. I did not understand their importance. My surgical blunders stay indelible in memory, evoking a mixture of shame and dread. Shame, because I did not think clearly and dread at the thought of a damaging outcome.

It was a week after we started work in Mokama. Devi Prasad, a middle-aged farmer, had agreed to have his gall bladder removed. He told me with a broad smile that he felt fortunate to be treated by the 'phoren doctor'. The surgery went well and everyone was pleased. So was I.

As it turned out, the self-congratulatory mood was unwarranted. Devi Prasad had been shifted to his bed in the general ward after recovering from the anaesthetic. Not long afterwards the nurse came to tell me that his blood pressure had gone down despite the rapid infusion of fluids.

'Must be the pethidine I gave him for pain,' the anaesthetist said. I felt reassured. Pethidine is an effective pain-relieving drug but it also lowers blood pressure.

Three hours later it was still low and falling steadily. The pulse was fast and feeble; his tongue, pale. Could it be internal haemorrhage? But how? I stood by his bedside in the male surgical general ward which had a little over thirty patients and tried to think back, *into* the abdomen. I had taken all the possible precautions...hadn't I? But just in case...* On reopening the still-raw, just-sutured incision, I was greeted by the sight of blood welling up inside the abdomen. The ligature I had placed around the artery supplying blood to the gall bladder had slipped and it was pumping blood. There were some tense

*Ultrasound scanning was at least a decade away, so the only option was to take him back to the operating theatre and have a look inside.

moments while I struggled to get hold of the bleeder and secure it with double ligatures. The incident taught me to always check the gall-bladder bed one last time before closing the wound. I felt grateful to that marvel called intuition which goaded me to reopen the wound, to the watchful nurse who had detected the problem and alerted me and to everyone present in the operating theatre for helping me see it through. The importance of team-work is driven home in such critical situations.

*

The hospital had free Sunday clinics for leprosy patients: a desk, two chairs and a stool would be placed on the open ground in front of the hospital. Patients would begin to come as early as seven in the morning. Leprosy can strike anyone, but is largely a disease of the destitute. History and literature offer lasting imagery of the suffering, deformities, humiliation and mental anguish caused by it. A successful cure came only in the 1960s. The hospital in Mokama offered treatment free of cost. Tuberculosis was, and still is, more rampant. The lungs, gut, skin, lymph nodes, eye, ear, brain, kidney, bone, breast, spine—it spares no part of the body. The results of correct treatment (surgery and or medicines) are excellent. Cholera is a constant visitor to village fairs and religious festivities. The furious outpouring of fluids and salts in the form of 'rice-water stools' can be fatal if untreated, and death can occur in a matter of hours. Cholera outbreaks were frequent in Bihar. The hospital had a 'cholera routine' during such epidemics when entire wards filled up with patients. I saw my first of several cases of diphtheria and tetanus in Mokama. Diphtheria was more amenable to treatment, when seen early. I don't think we saved a single case of tetanus which infected newborns whose umbilical stump had been sealed with cowdung, a trusted antiseptic in Bihar.

*

Operating on injuries borne out of criminal violence was not central to my work but they were incessant, difficult and exhausting. Burns were as common as gunshot injuries, and more tragic. Invariably they were reported to have resulted from the accidental bursting of a stove. Why were the victims of burns young, married women every time and why did the stove *not* burst when an unmarried daughter of the house or an older woman cooked? Once in a while, a baby fell into a vessel of boiling water and during Diwali kids got injured by firecrackers. Only once did I see a man who had suffered burns, and they were minor.

Burns patients were isolated in a five-bedded ward to effectively replace lost body fluids and salts, dress and excise wounds, transfer blood and do skin grafts. The agony from denuded nerve endings needed round-the-clock medication. Burns treatment takes up a lot of time. After the initial days of intravenous fluids and blood, many patients need surgical excision of dead tissue and skin grafting. Young women who recovered from burns that had been inflicted on them would, in all likelihood, have to return to the same wretched household.

Sudha was carried into the clinic by her brother and placed on the examination couch. Even in that position you could tell that she was tall—with a ready smile and bold voice. She had suffered the burns seven years ago, a few months after her marriage when she was seventeen. Burst stove. She survived the burns, registered a case against her husband and in-laws and saw them go to prison. Deep burns had scarred her perineum and lower limbs, leaving her with severely deformed knees folded up against her thighs due to insufficient treatment. The perineal insult meant that she would never have a normal married life, or bear children.

'What can we do for you?' I asked, barely able to hide my misgivings. It seemed a hopeless case.

'I want to stand on my feet and walk. Whatever it takes, I'm willing to pay.' She showed me a thick bundle of notes.

I suggested she go to Patna or Calcutta where she would have a better chance. Sudha said she had entrusted her faith to this hospital and that was that. The multiple surgeries, the excisions and skin graft took six weeks of endurance. Even during the treatment, I often wished she would get frustrated and go elsewhere. But Sudha remained steadfast. Somewhere along the way, her resolve and confidence became mine. The result was reasonably good. The knees were not fully straight and her gait was stiff, like that of an old woman. She needed crutches. But walk she did.

I asked Sudha if she feared for her life. What if her husband came after her once his prison term was over? I can well recollect the Bihari lilt of her voice: 'Bataaiey Daaktar Saab... darr ke jeene se kuch faida hai?' Is living in fear of any use?

*

Looking through some old notebooks I found a record of the surgical cases I had undertaken in Mokama. The twelve-month list gives me a fair idea of the bleakness and the turmoil of violence. There would be quiet periods when it would mock us by its absence so much so that there would be time to stroll on the terrace above our living quarters. Here on clear nights the stars were our nearest neighbours. These were moments of restful quiet, while all the time, somewhere a country-gun was being oiled and readied.

Gun battles happened most often between criminal gangs who made a living out of extortions, abductions, drug transactions and killings to settle political or personal grudges. The weapon used to be the country gun, or the 'blunderbuss': an old-fashioned gun with a short musket, a fan-shaped muzzle and wide bore made to spray the pellets at close range. In killing, the criminals rarely blundered and I saw the outcome once too often. I entered the world of criminals without any warning. There was no preparatory course, no advisory caveat that came with the job. Except that you do not give up on any patient.

Violent and grave injuries could not be wished away to another hospital; the nearest, in Patna, was 90 kilometres away. The initial fear and dismay gave way to a feeling of wonder, and the quiet joy of entering the cramped operating room day after day or night, to wash and scrub and prepare to sew lacerated flesh, fix fragmented bone and tremblingly suture pulsing vessels and tubes so torn up that mud, sand, grass and bits of metal oozed out with the material of living substance. And all I had to do was save a life; believe that this teenager, who chose to be a gun-toting criminal, must breathe, his blood must flow in smooth, predetermined channels, the skin must stay warm, his eyes must open and the limbs must move. Bodies torn open by bullets are difficult to repair. Through the night hours we tracked the bullets inside muscle, bone, kidney, stomach and intestine, with the smell of melted metal mocking the efforts of our 'bed' be-dragged team. Ninety per cent of gunshot injuries came after midnight.

As one of a team of ant-workers, all fifty kilos of me had to stay bent under the stern blue lights, sweating rivers of concentration until at last I could look at Sister Margaret Mary, the anaesthetist at the head-end of the operating table, and see something flicker in her eyes. A faint smile of relief would crease my mask; I would straighten my back just a little, knowing that my neck will start to hurt even more in a while. My clothes would hold me in a wet and bloody embrace. Oh heck. Bernadette would soon take care of the routine post-operative matters, the rest of us could unlock our joints, pull down the sweaty masks and reach for coffee. The change of clothes could wait.

'Doctor, will you check his lungs—I can't hear breath sounds on the right side.'

Half an hour of anxiety later, coffee. There were instances

when I thought we were done and that we had done well, the patient having been shifted from the OT stretcher to the ward stretcher, when the anaesthetist would shout, 'Cardiac arrest!' and half an hour of failed resuscitation later, I would go out to meet the fretful relatives to say what no surgeon wants to say and no relative wants to hear: 'I'm sorry…'

The toll had been paid. But there was more to come. Always, there is more coming. The body can only assume a state of semi-rest, which is also fine. I was only twenty-eight.

An average of one gunshot wound every six or seven days was normal. Other acts of violent crime—an assortment of deadly wounds from bows-and-arrows, scuffles with knives, injuries from country bombs—provided the piquancy. It was not yet noon one day when a young man was wheeled in to my clinic ahead of others who waited.

'Kya hua?' I was a trifle annoyed, for the young man appeared quite normal. He looked at me with unblinking eyes, lifted a hand and moved aside the scarf covering his neck. A neat cut, like a surgical incision, had laid open his wind-pipe. A homicidal tracheostomy, with the voice-box damaged? No wonder he was speech-less. Following surgery he was in hospital for a couple of weeks while the wounds healed and he regained his voice.

I was curious about the injury and asked him how he had come by the wound. 'Chhath se girgaya.' Fell off the roof, he said, without any hesitation.

A victim who survives violence is her or his own best witness. Telling the truth, however, can be just too dicey: luck does not hold out every time. This, every Bihari knows.

*

The nurses were from that region down south where getting ahead in life is as much a uniting principle as the eating of fish and coconut and the wearing of the simple white mundu.

Nursing is an unusual job demanding emotional strength and disciplined skills. Fresh out of Kerala high schools, the girls had to contend with north Indian summers and intense winters, language difficulties, nightshifts and long hours of work. Most of them would go back to live within the constructs of a patriarchal society where good job prospects and the strength of character help women to live with dignity. The nuns understood this. For the first three months the nursing students were taught the values of decorum, deportment, and the ability to communicate in Hindi and English.

Nutritious food was provided by the hospital kitchen; the girls played shuttle and throw-ball, watched movies on Sunday evenings, partook in music and dance competitions. I don't think they missed their homes very much. With their hard-driven need to excel, these Malayali girls showed the way to those from Bengal, Assam, Mizoram and Meghalaya, and very rarely from Bihar itself, where the idea of attending to the sick—especially men—was held to be unsuitable for young girls. Nursing has changed this concept. Nursing schools, particularly those run by Christian institutions, have played a huge role in the upliftment of nurses. They are the single largest group of educated female professionals in our country: the trend-setters of women's liberation.

For the nurses as much as doctors, the dynamics of violence, oppression and poverty so clearly seen in Mokama were instructive; and at times just too much. An eighty-year-old American who lived much of his priestly life in Mokama was shot and killed by miscreants who barged into his room at the seminary and pumped him with bullets. Reason: the diesel-generator from the monastery had been stolen and the priest had confronted some local youths. He knew they were the culprits and he told them that if they returned the generator he would not go to the police. They preferred an easier settlement of scores.

One afternoon, a couple of student nurses noticed a boy of about eleven or twelve loitering near the hospital. He looked very ill and they brought him in. His right arm was covered in sores, blistered and swollen from fingertips to armpit. He was febrile and restless. The infection went deep, with dead and dying muscle hanging loose, like overcooked meat. He wouldn't say what happened, only that he worked for some big person along with other boys. They 'made things'.

What things?

He would not say.

The boy had no visitors. The arm healed after weeks of treatment but it looked like he would lose two fingers rendered useless by the infection. When he was told, he shook his violently. No! Next morning, his bed was empty. He had run away. Much later we learned that he had been working in a home-based factory that made fire-crackers. Of what kind, I wonder.

At one particular, practical level a hospital is but a factory that repairs damaged or malfunctioning 'items' and attempts to make them as near normal as possible. It hums with the busy-ness of a factory. The nuns have a special gift for nursing the sick, (the priests are more suited for the seminary and its various activities.) The pharmacy, laboratory, office, finance department, stores, kitchen, nursing school and the wards came under the sharp eye of nuns trained in specific fields, three of them being doctors. The local men and women were trained as ward-clerks, office assistants, nurse-aides, cleaners, cooks and gardeners. You must see the plight of the poor and the landless of Bihar to understand the significance of such uplift. One frequently hears derisive comments about missionaries enticing the poor into Christianity. But this change of religion, more often than not, equips them with education and good health. Moreover, they become part of a thought and faith system where they are no longer treated as lesser human beings because of an accident of birth.

13

Speaking of Krishna...

When we moved from Mokama in Bihar to Vrindavan in Uttar Pradesh, we thought that work would be, well—more peaceful. We spent several years at a hospital in Vrindavan run by the Ramakrishna Mission. Vrindavan is in Mathura district, on the eastern banks of the Yamuna. Religion and folklore infuse this little town with a distinctive flavour. Krishna is believed to have spent his childhood and youth in Vrindavan herding cows, playing the flute, romping with the gopis and vanquishing evil. He is one of the most colourful religious representations of the Almighty to have ignited the minds of poets, artists and musicians.* Here shrunken Bengali widows chant bhajans in the temples to earn their twelve-hourly victuals of rice and daal; ash-smeared sadhus armed with tridents weave through the vegetable markets. Janmashtami, the day of Krishna's birth, stretches into a week-long carnival when locals who live elsewhere hasten home to join in the festivities.

Given the eccentric nature of the town where ancient temples rub shoulders with garish neo-architecture, the unflappably staid hospital appeared something of a novelty. Within the five-acre campus are hospital buildings, the monastery, mandir and

---

*Sur Das, Tulsi Das and the Sufi poet Amir Khusro composed in the local braj basha. (Vraja basha became braj basha; Bengalis who predominate the area do not use the labio-dental apposition which produces the sound va.)

living quarters for doctors and staff. The monastery is a circular building with an inner courtyard and living quarters for the monks and trainee brahmacharis; the softly contoured mandir with pink walls had managed to escape religious extravagance. In the 1980s when we joined, dozens of cows were being reared at the ashram and milk was plentiful. The kitchen provided admitted patients with food; doctors and staff could choose to eat in the long dining room of the monastery, along with the resident monks. You sat on the floor and ate from steel thalis that you washed yourself. The fastidiously nurtured garden, the fields of wheat, the tamarind and Asoka trees provided a soft and tranquil ambience.

The wards were large, the operating theatre well-designed and lavish by rural standards. The seven or eight doctors who staffed the hospital were used to getting by with complete disregard for discipline. The surgeon and his two lackey ward-boys had more or less high-jacked the system. A few retired doctors did 'honorary' work while fulfilling their religious obligations with regular visits to the mandir. They were good people but largely self-serving, and content to have housing, food, security and medical benefits in exchange for the lightest of work.

The only exception to this devout bunch was the physician: a Hindi-speaking Welshman who lived by the message of the Sermon on the Mount and the words of Swami Vivekananda. His ward rounds would begin at six every morning. By half-past seven when the rest of us trooped in, he would be in the nurses' duty room, writing patient-records in his distinctive scrawl or speaking to an anxious relative. In sizzling summer months Dr Jones would wear his white coat over his vest, revealing the flare of heat rash on pink skin. He served the local people for over thirty years, until the end of his working life.

The surgeon was well-groomed, fortyish and elusive; he treated me with dismissive courtesy. The anaesthetist was polite but uncommunicative. My first day inside the operating theatre was awkward, to say the least. The surgeon, having changed into the grey pant-and-shirt theatre uniform, walked in holding a burning cigarette between his fingers. He leaned over the operating table to watch Lakhan, the ward boy, remove a steel rod from a patient with a hip fracture; having snapped out instructions, the surgeon headed for the doctor's room to smoke another cigarette. Then the anaesthetist came in to announce that the next case—a hernia—would be delayed because the wife was yet to sign the consent form for surgery. We drank tea and made small talk until the patient was wheeled in. Just then the matron peeped with a request from some friend of the surgeon who wanted to speak to him whereby he vanished for some twenty minutes. In the meantime, the anaesthetist put the patient to sleep and Lakhan scrubbed up, cleaned and draped the operation site. This was routine. The ward boy would assist the surgeon, do minor surgical procedures and finish the suturing for his boss. He too was known as 'daacter saab'.

The nurses were Malayalis, every one of them, and had passed or failed tenth standard. The only nursing they knew they had learned from the matron, a motherly queen bee, with the knowingness of a seasoned housewife. It led to parts of the hospital resembling a kitchen: nurses were allowed to warm their food on the stove meant for boiling the glass syringes and needles. If a doctor went to the wards at certain hours, the nurses would gladly offer to make tea. Patients' attenders waited their turn to cook dalia and boil milk. The pharmacy was chaotic: a mile-long room in the basement with one befuddled swami in charge. On his frail shoulders fell the responsibility of managing stocks, indents, supplies, sales and bills. Whenever I tried to speak to him about the problems in the pharmacy, I saw the simmering panic in his eyes and toned down my grievances. Poor man, his real passion was music. He sang bhajans, some of them his own compositions, in the mandir every evening. The music must have worked like a sort of self-therapy for this unobtrusive sadhu who had to cope with medicinal matters that were way beyond him. The laboratory was managed by a dour-looking doctor attired in a starched dhoti and shirt, with a taciturnity which suited his daily routine of sticking needles into arms, drawing blood, looking into a microscope, shaking test tubes and writing reports. I never saw him smile or even look cheerful; but he was meticulous, and competent.

Not having professional experience themselves, the swamis were powerless to handle the wayward doctors and staff. They atoned for this weakness with a foolproof accounting system which was remarkably good. Two swamis, two novice brahmacharis and an assistant worked at the office which resounded with the comforting din of typewriters. Bills were worked out, payments documented, accounts maintained and audited, salaries paid on time. It made up in some small way for the unruliness and disarray in other parts of the hospital.

We struggled to adjust. The hospital in Mokama with its discipline, cleanliness and nursing care was easier to work in. Here, we were frustrated and unhappy. One morning I went into the Head Swami's office—a small room overfilled with books, papers and tiers of files held together with red string and stacked on tall shelves. There was just enough space for a visitor to sit across from his desk.

'You should not have employed us,' I blurted, hotly. 'We're qualified doctors, and here you don't even have qualified nurses.' I said something about the sun's chariot and the six horses, without making much sense. 'Why don't you get quacks instead? Run your hospital exactly as you please. We're quitting.'

The Head Swami was a strong boulder of a man from Bengal and had been a pilot in the air force before joining the monastery. He looked at me across the desk, the spectacled face was expressionless.

'Doctore,' he said, sweetly. 'Now that you know how difficult it is to run a hospital here, please be kind enough to put your experience into practice. Improve it. I will give all the help you need.'

'I—I'm a doctor,' I gulped. 'It's not my job—'

'Six horses, you said, doctore. Pulling together. I know. I understand. Help us to set it right. You will have two hundred per cent support from me.'

I saw the cunning twinkle in his eyes and knew I had met an astute and intelligent man. He had no need of my brashness, what he needed were doctors he could trust. He had put me in my place, not with rude retaliation, but with the offer of a chance for a rethink before quitting. How clever, and how kind. I went home to talk about it with my husband. We decided to stay.

From the little office where he sat all day, the swami kept track of the goings-on in the rest of the hospital. He had a trusted deputy, a genial swami who spent most of his working hours in the wards, talking to the sick and answering their ceaseless queries. The hospital was so very affordable, but in Vrindavan, it was a matter of principle to ask for a discount. Women wrung their hands and men fell at the feet of the swami, pleading him to bring the negligible hospital fees down a few notches.

A chilly November morning a couple of days after my outburst in the office, all of us who worked at the hospital, kitchen, monastery, mandir and garden were asked to gather at the hospital entrance. An odd mix of about sixty people: doctors in white coats, nurses in sari-uniforms; the matron with the wide red belt around her maternal waist, and the starched triangle banner of a cap; ward boys, monks and brahmacharis from the office; the cleaners, Vichitra the gardener, Kishan the cowherd, Fakira the watchman and the edentulous, Gandhi-cap-wearing Janu Mama who cleaned the toilets in the houses within the compound. The Head Swami explained in his Bangla-accented Hindi that he proposed to bring about certain changes in the hospital. It required absolute discipline and proper conduct from every one of us.

'This hospital is like the Sun God, sitting astride his chariot and our Guruji is the charioteer.' He gave me a quick glance of acknowledgement. 'We, that is doctors, swamis, nurses, staff, this-one-that-one-everyone represent the six horses of the Sun. *Hraam, Hreem, Hroom, Hrain, Hroum, Hraha* are the horses which ensure that the sun journeys as per the Eternal Law. Likewise, from now on we move together in one direction, with one purpose.'

I think to most of us, he looked every bit as determined as the sun.

Excessive words perhaps, but from then on every morning the Head Swami appeared at that very spot on the topmost steps that led to the hospital. He issued commands. Little did he expect the reaction of the staff to this imposition of discipline. Long used to a casual manner of work, most of the doctors and nurses were unhappy. We, the two new doctors, were the interlopers trying to impose a foreign style of running the hospital. Some adjusted, others left and a few had to go. The surgeon, the anaesthetist, the matron and a ward boy set up practice outside the hospital. Eight nurses and a few of the other staff struck work. It was a very difficult time, and for a while there were the occasional riotous scenes in the hospital. Indiscipline was not the only problem: one doctor was fired for assaulting a nurse; an office clerk was ticked off for writing romantic missives to a lady doctor and knocking on her doors at all hours to proclaim his undying love. He was probably harmless, but the poor man was told to pack up and marched off through the gates, carrying a small tin trunk of his possessions.*

The hospital had functioned all along with the belief that treating the sick was an act of kindness and charity, like the giving of alms. This belief persists in many religious and other well-meaning institutions. Even when done with the best of intentions, such free treatment eventually becomes a soulless service. The giver takes on the role of a superior being, some sort of god before whom the receiver stoops with gratitude. Free treatment is sometimes essential—as in times of major disasters, or some major personal catastrophe which results in utter destitution. And even so, the giver, be it a doctor, a priest, a wealthy man or a corporate house, has no business to feel superior or deliver it as an act of piety. The Head Swami was sporting enough to listen to our arguments. He then used his wisdom to do what was necessary to better organize the hospital.

The pharmacy was resurrected and a physiotherapy department was set up. Weekly clinical meetings were held where doctors could meet and discuss their patients. We mustered up the courage—no, the audacity—to set up a nursing school. After weeks of discussion and planning, an advertisement was placed in a newspaper in Kerala (where else?) calling for applications. Ten girls thus selected arrived, each with a tin trunk of possessions. Along with a nursing instructor (a retired teacher from Mangalore), some of us doctors were entrusted with the task of training them. We did so in earnest, teaching Anatomy, Physiology, Nursing Arts and the clinical subjects as set by the nursing curriculum and also English and

---

*None of the difficulties prepared any of us for the bludgeoning of a pharmacy assistant by his friend over a tiff regarding a nurse. It happened one hot afternoon. The killer took a hammer to the head of his friend as he reclined in bed reading the papers, walked out of the room, bolting the door after him, washed his hands at a sink and left through the hospital gates, never to be seen again. The victim died on the operating table the same night.

Hindi. For me, it was a great way to learn nursing techniques. (There are nine ways of bed-making, did you know?)

The tutor, a Mangalore Catholic, was as austere and disciplined as any swami and matched them in earnestness. Every evening at sundown when evening prayers and aarti were held at the mandir, a small bunch of Catholic nursing students gathered in Ms Alva's room for prayers. It seems a remarkable thing now, but in those days in Uttar Pradesh we lived in comfortable harmony with people of different religious faiths.

The hospital services were no longer free but still, cheaper than peanuts. A bed in the general ward cost two rupees a day, with food. The outpatient fee was half-a-rupee, with blood, urine, stool and sputum examinations taken care of. Patients came bearing 'samples' in little newspaper-wrapped bottles, or a matchbox.*

At the outpatient clinic, thirty patients were all I could handle in a day. Twenty-nine of those thirty were rural and small-town folk from Govardhan, Nandagaon, Hathras or Kosi and the neighbouring villages. They could manage the rock-bottom rates of the hospital. The very sick were brought in on makeshift stretchers, or ferried across the Yamuna. A few times a week, some well-to-do owner of a mithai shop or an army man unhappy with the military hospital in Mathura or a holy person of comfortable means would turn up. I was often startled by humbly clad purveyors of religion who uncovered their bodies to reveal dangerous secrets. The widows of Vrindavan, most of them discarded in the land of God, were treated free. Uniformly small, shrivelled, shaven, toothless and bent over with physical and nutritional fatigue and clad in coarse white, they were like shadows with all the joy of life knocked out of them. With names like Govardhan Dasi, Gokul Dasi, Radha

---

*There is this joke about a patient who anxiously asks the doctor how he should bring a sample of his stool and the doctor snaps, 'Bring it in a dalda tin.' And that's what the man did.

Devi, Vrindavan Maayi—they were a persistent and invisible presence on the streets, making their way in the scorching heat to some temple to chant all day just to be able to eat. Their weakened bones were susceptible to fractures. In the wards, they were the only patients who did not complain.

The mandir held prayers in the early morning and just before sunset. The temple bells and the gentle melody of prayer floated through the corridors and into the operating theatre where we worked during the day and very often at night. In spite of the many changes in the hospital, religion held its own. Trouble of every description could be explained away as fate, destiny, or sins committed in one's previous birth. The decision to operate on a critical case in emergency situations was made right there on the corridor outside the wards, with the patient still on the stretcher. The two people I had to consult before deciding on surgery were the anaesthetist, and the deputy swami who hovered in the background, listening and watching as we shouted orders, set up drips, undid soaked clothing and spoke to relatives. The cases we saw were very varied. The proximity of Vrindavan to Agra and Delhi resulted in a confusing mix of rural fixity and urban restlessness. The people were noisy, demanding, unreasonable and truculent, or bound by archaic customs; they were quick to get worked up over imagined problems: the risk-versus-safety factor, an auspicious time, the sentiments, the disfavour of scheming relatives, religious pedants…all of it created a perpetual buzz of apprehension. I would be screamed at now and then, and I would scream back. Occasionally a brawl of some sort ensued but thanks to the ever-composed swami, it simmered down quickly.

Religion apart, the town was devoid of attractions. The movie theatres were in Mathura, 14 kilometres away and so were the schools, and shops where you could buy a blouse-piece or a sari, a bottle of Nescafe or Bournvita. We travelled in overloaded buses, cycle-rickshaws or our own Bajaj two-wheeler. I had my hair cut in an upstairs room where a girl just out of school snipped and sheared, with her mother directing her every move: '...a little bit here...that's it, a little more. That's too much! Ullu! Now you have to clip it off the other side too...' An hour-long exertion for the girl and five rupees of my money later, I would come down the stairs to hear comments like, 'You'll not need a haircut for another year.'

In my early days in Vrindavan, I experienced what can be best described as an 'age-and-gender-issue'. The hardy north-Indian farmers would look at me, mutter and frown and shaking their heads, take the patient away. A young female surgeon was all wrong. For some months I was mistaken for an assistant to some worthy male superior somewhere inside the operating theatre brooding over his next surgical feat. The two ward boys, being male, were believed to be higher up the ladder than me. Once, a week or so after operating on a young man to remove a ruptured spleen, I was about to show a trainee nurse how to remove the sutures when the patient said, 'I want daakter saab to do it,' and pointed to one of the ward boys. 'I'm the doctor,' I said, and then realizing how feeble my case must look, left it to daakter saab.

North Indian summers are cruel. Working hours were from half-past-seven in the morning till one for lunch-cum-collapse and then again till five, six or whenever. We did not work by the clock, except at the start of day after which, time ceased to exist. Ward rounds, seeing new patients, operating, arguing with relatives—are all part of hospital life. A concerned relative must be spoken to, but a bunch of them pressing forward with questions can be difficult. Among them were also some who had other questions: 'Tera byah haigo kaah? (Are you married?), followed by 'Gharkon-kon hai re?' (Who are the people at home?) and if you say 'husband and I', there will be sorrowful exclamations, fervently offered prayers and exhortations to visit one or other of the famed sadhus/sadhwinis of Vrindavan (Mouni baba, Pagla Baba, Anand Mai…)

It was a marvellous job. Much of the credit for our success with many difficult cases goes to my husband who had, by then, switched to anaesthesia. He also had exceptional organizational and administrative skills which the hospital management could make use of. Countless were the instances when he pulled a patient out of danger using the most ingenious methods. He imposed stringent discipline on everyone he worked with. I admired him, but on rare occasions our egos clashed and one of us stepped back to maintain peace. Taking care of the 'head-end' of a patient while the surgeon performs her task is a skill that demands expertise, quick reflexes and equanimity. The competence of the anaesthetist is crucial for surgery. If I have done anything worthy as a surgeon in all these years, it is thanks to my anaesthetists.

Working without a mentor revealed the deficiencies in my knowledge. My experience was entirely based on what I had learnt from my teachers, books, colleagues and training courses. Successful rural practitioners have to acquire wide-ranging skills. Many surgeons work without the help of a physician to deal with medical problems. He treats the diabetic foot after getting the patient out of her keto-acidosis which is a serious complication of diabetes; he monitors the cardiac status, hypertension and asthma, helps women through safe pregnancies, does urgent Caesareans, repairs tendons, sets fractures, manages tuberculosis, rheumatoid arthritis and Parkinson. All this and much more get done in our lesser-known hospitals. In today's rural practice it has become a little easier to get the advice of fellow-surgeons and specialists through email or the phone. Specialists, particularly those who were colleagues and have top experience in their fields, often go out of their way to help solve a difficult case. Technology, when used prudently, is of enormous help in the exchange of ideas and knowledge.

Looking back, I see myself evolving as a surgeon during my years in Vrindavan. In UK most of the time we operated under perfect conditions and the variety was nowhere as wide as in India. After the initial period of training, the weekly operating lists became predictable and dull. How many hernias, varicose veins, gall bladders and stomach ulcers can one do with any excitement? The dour, law-abiding British were obedient patients. The only problem was that most of them were well-muscled or obese. The surgeon had to labour through inches of abdominal fat before reaching muscle, and then enter the operative site. The wiry women and hardy men of our villages are much easier to work on.

I loved the unpredictability and the volatile madness of Vrindavan, the gullibility of faith, the eye-popping images of advanced disease and even the piquant arguments which raged in the hospital corridors. These and other features of my work rounded off my surgical training. Excitement of the surgical sort were never far away. Volvulus or ('twisted gut' where several feet of intestine get twisted around the pedicle, causing the affected loops of bowel to strangulate), diverticuli (small polyp-like protuberances of the gut that can bleed or get infected), intussusception (where a loop of bowel plunges into its own lumen, causing a blockage) are some of the emergency abdominal surgeries which are as exciting as they are taxing. There were daily duels with broken bones, bleeding or inverted uteruses, bicornuate or two-horned uterus (which I saw in a twin pregnancy where the twins had private cubicles!) the phlegmon (abscess), the bubo (a syphilitic lymph node), the split skull, the pulped malarial spleen, the liver gashed and gut in tatters; the maggots, worms, bacteria and viruses. The known and the unknown, the chilling, fantabulous, near-apocryphal deviations from normal. You cannot refuse a patient with a fungating cancer of the penis or a young woman with a hideous hemangioma of her eyelid just because it is your first encounter with the disease. The Agra Medical College and the hospitals in Delhi were accessible to only a few who could afford to go. The rural surgeon ('Jajjan' Madam in my case) must find ways to manage. Everything that appears on the plate is yours to handle with the knife, fork and spoon.*

There was independence in work, even when I *wanted* to be dependent. I came to rely on the *British Medical Journal* (BMJ) to keep myself updated, along with *The Annals of the Royal College of Surgeons*, which was my favourite for content and style. The Indian edition of the BMJ served well for years until its publication was stopped, leaving me deprived of a perfect teacher. For a few years when we were in Vrindavan, we received a surgical journal, the cyclostyled copies of which were sent free. Each instalment dealt with a specific subject, with expert opinion and operative steps described in lucid style. I learnt many valuable surgical lessons through this journal.

But the books were my saviours. Never did a pre-op day pass when I did not pore over *Grant's Atlas of Anatomy* or one of the several surgical books in preparation for a case. The unexpected intra-operative problem becomes the scissor's edge poised over a patient's life. The only option for a surgeon is to win. How many times have I stood with wads of gauze pressed over a pumping vessel, fighting down panic, combining patience with judgement on when to take that pressure away and go after the bleeder, clamp, ligate and when the bleeding finally stops, looked up and seen the relieved faces around me! The patient sleeps through it and the relatives waiting outside the theatre doors need only know the finish.

In six years, we attained a level of efficiency which pleases me. Our small team of five doctors held clinical meetings on Saturday afternoons in a poky little room opposite the

---

*No exaggeration here, I have used serving spoons to scoop out pus from deep inside the pelvic basin and from an abscess cavity hiding behind the liver when power failure rendered the suction machine useless.

operating theatre. Rare and interesting cases were presented in turn; we discussed the dangers of antibiotic-overuse, agreed and disagreed. As a result, the routine of obliging patients with injections or the glucose 'drip' without proper justification was stopped. Patients seeking quick relief were unhappy. A painful poke or a bottle dripping its noble contents into your bloodstream feels like something vital is being done. Injections were very popular; there was an Injection Room in the outpatient department where hundred or more eager patients waited their turn every day. When this changed, patients were aghast. What? No *sooyi?* This hospital is looting our money, handing over coloured pills, fit only to chuck in the nulla…

*

Delhi was three hours by bus or train, and we went a couple of times every year. A room for two in Karol Bagh cost fifty bucks, which was affordable if we made do with inexpensive and delicious street-food. During one such train journey I read that a dangerous sexually transmitted disease had been detected in the US. It had first appeared in parts of Central Africa and then spread westward. The disease was apparently far removed from our shores but it was progressive and fatal; the risks were real. All of Delhi was agog; in the campus of a college we happened to visit, the students were being cautioned about the dangers of sexual encounters; mothers sighed with new-found despair. The terms HIV and AIDS were being used everywhere with little understanding and a lot of confusion. Dissatisfied with my own lack of understanding, I spent the best part of several months piecing it all together until I felt confident to speak about it at the weekly clinical meeting.

The Human Immunodeficiency Virus (HIV) had apparently been around for a few hundred years, thriving in certain species of chimpanzees, apes and monkeys. Western colonizers hunting in the wilds of Central Africa would skin or cut up bush-meat with help from the natives who worked with them. The virus probably entered humans through minor cuts and abrasions on their hands, since any raw surface or wound can allow access to the virus. The other risk was the custom of female circumcision and sexual activity in young girls, as also prostitution and homosexuality. Like syphilis some centuries earlier, this deadly virus spread through sexual partners, through blood transfusions, and to the newborn of an infected mother during its last moments of passage through the birth canal. At our weekly meeting, a few of my colleagues protested strongly when I said that it would soon reach India and cause havoc unknown since the days of the plague and smallpox. 'You are talking about a disease which affects sexually promiscuous, immoral societies,' said one of the doctors. 'There is little danger of it coming to India.'

We had an argument. I survived his scowling countenance until the first case was diagnosed in a laboratory in Madras and any complacence about our sexual value-system was shot to pieces.

*

It must have been the affable nature of the swamis which emboldened me to treat them as friends. There were many among them who could take a joke. To be humourless *and* religious can be a dreadful thing. My best friend was the deputy. He would listen to my rants with much politeness; at times a smile would engulf his face, or he would throw back his head and laugh. I often came away feeling that I had spoken out of ignorance. Even so, being young and brazen, I was keen to air my views and hold fast to my convictions: it was standard practice in Vrindavan to address a swami as 'Maharaj', and to touch his feet in greeting. I stuck to 'Swamiji' and never touched any feet. I was set upon by wives of doctors and a few other ladies who entreated me to follow tradition, at first sweetly and then with the belligerence of too much faith. I was also told it would be good if I went to the mandir every evening for the aarti. On one occasion when the president of Ramakrishna Mission visited the hospital, it was made clear that everyone would touch his feet and receive blessings. We lined up in a long queue. The saintly old swami acknowledged my namaste with a warm smile. Certain customs are meant to be broken.

In Vrindavan I discovered that rural surgery would be my specialization. Distancing oneself from city lights does not mean the mind should turn as dim as the lights in a village. Moreover, the skies are clear, the stars are alive and for several days every month I get to read by moonlight. Life is perhaps less complicated. Villagers who come to the hospital are hardy and eat simple food. Their bodies are less corrupted by drug overuse and misuse, less violated by multiple investigations and confusing specialist opinions. They tend to keep loyalties. If I do a hernia repair on the husband, it is likely that his wife will approach me for her hysterectomy and when the son busts his ankle, I'm expected to set it right.

A rural doctor enjoys the touching hospitality that is typical to rural societies: complimentary tea and samosas for the daakter at the cinema while watching a B-grade Hindi film or a Bhojpuri blockbuster, bunches of bananas, papaya or pumpkin and seasonal homemade delicacies wrapped in newspaper. You brace yourself to cope with their curiosity too, and curiosity never died down. 'How many children do you have? One! A girl! Hai Ram!' they would say. Native remedies abounded: a rejuvenating tonic made of unshelled raw eggs; coffee powder to stem bleeding; 'rat-ear-leaf' for diabetes; cowdung or bandar-ka-tatti for open wounds.

The imposing ISKCON temple built of pink sandstone was a more recent addition to the profusion of temples dating back to the 8th century. The Krishna Consciousness movement is an aggressively pious edition of religion favoured by Western zealots who use missionary fervour to propagate a brand of brahminical Hinduism propounded by Swami Prabhupadananda. ISKCON maintains its own gurukul for training little boys, mostly European. Their mothers, draped in saffron saris, sweep the temple courtyards and their well-muscled fathers officiate at the temple, beat drums, dance and sing devotional songs. To our eyes, the gaudiness of it was blinding and offensive. We went to the ISKCON temple as spectators, sipped kullads of cardamom tea in a tea-stall opposite and came away with the delicious prasadam distributed free at the temple.

I paid for my small act of wickedness by being pincered by religiosity for a while: having operated on a nine-year-old German lad for a burst appendix, I was cornered by his father and spoken to. I listened with politeness and smiled evasively when he solicited my serious commitment to god and bhakti; I begged off by saying that I had too much to do. He wrote letters—page after page after page of esoteric devotional rant—and then one afternoon he came home, steely blue eyes blazing with manic belief. My endurance had worn thin by then and I blurted that I did not need to be 'converted' to Hindu religion or any religion, and least of all, by a convert. He spewed out a few rude-sounding German words and walked out, slamming the door.

The monks in Vrindavan and the nuns in Bihar abrogated the caste system with all sincerity. But conditioned to its insidious influences, they sometimes fell short. On the birthday of Swami Vivekananda, the garden space of the hospital would be thrown open to many hundreds for a sumptuous meal. It was a much-awaited ritual, an opportunity for the swamis and hospital staff to mingle with the people of Vrindavan. During this moving spectacle of universal compassion, the lower castes were fed a little distance away from the rest. Why?

'People will not accept,' said one of the swamis.

In Mokama, at an interview for junior doctors, the sister in charge of administration asked each applicant his caste. I objected. 'We prefer doctors from lower castes,' she explained to me. 'Job opportunities of this sort are limited for them, which means they are less likely to quit the job too soon.' It also meant they would be less demanding of salary hikes and perquisites.

Religion, religiosity, crookery and the sublime joys of a working life. Engulfed by confusing traditions, I took up cudgels against all of it.

I also began to write.

14

City Lights

'It may seem a strange principle to enunciate as the very first requirement in a hospital that it should do the sick no harm.'—Florence Nightingale.

Between the previous chapter and this, lies the period when my first marriage soured and ended. It is a personal zone of unhappiness from which we both emerged and remade our lives. I am grateful for all the good that came during those years.

Vijay and I got married in 1994. We lived in the city of Madras where Vijay had a job at *The Hindu*. With a college friend's help, I found work in the surgical department of a five-storeyed private hospital with six hundred beds and all the major specialities. The boss—a surgeon—welcomed me effusively and offered a fair salary. The distinct change in my career made me nervous, but I assured myself that it was a chance to learn. Madras had long been known for its fine doctors and medical institutions. It just so happened that what I experienced was vastly different.

Everything in the hospital revolved around the boss. The mornings began with the team of doctors, assistants and interns waiting for him to arrive. We waited for hours: he came as late as noon, or before nine, or sometime in between, there was no telling when. A few days after I joined, he told me that I should stick to the female patients and not males. I was truly taken aback. Later, in emergency situations and high-risk cases, he broke his own rule and sent for me. His surgical judgement was so poor as to be embarrassing. If any assistant offered a suggestion, he would snap: 'I'm the boss here, I make the decisions.' I was reduced to assisting him in his innumerable goof-ups. He tried to inveigle me with the promise of a better salary, status and so on if I admitted more patients and took a more active part in bringing good returns to the hospital. One day I was in his clinic, listening to him boast about some surgery he planned to do when a man in his thirties hobbled in on crutches. An engineer working in Dubai, he had sustained a simple fracture of his heel bone six weeks ago. He was home on leave. Since he was free of pain, all he wanted was to know if he could start walking without crutches. The boss did a cursory examination of his foot and said, 'I think you should have an MRI to be hundred per cent sure that the bone has healed.'

The man thanked him effusively. 'The two doctors who treated me never suggested this,' he said. 'I'm happy I came to you.'

You cannot help patients who ask to be duped.

The general ward charges were Rs 750 a day.* The inmates were auto-rickshaw drivers, carpenters, painters, peons, porters and odd-job men. The question they asked repeatedly was, 'When will I be able to go home?' The hospital had a charitable wing which was a portion of the terrace roofed over with tin sheets. Imagine what is like for a patient to lie there in the 40 plus degrees Celsius summers of Madras. Extensive burns, gaping ulcers, non-healing wounds, the cirrhotic, the terminally ill, the consumptive (affected by tuberculosis) and the cachectic

---

*A staggering amount by the standards I was used to. Twenty years later, general ward beds in rural hospitals range from Rs 30 to Rs 50 a day. Government hospital beds of course come free.

(extremely emaciated) languished in the unmerciful heat—a few feet of cemented brick walls and ceramic floors separating them from the air-conditioned comforts of rooms below. No patient opted for this free ward, those who had neither money nor the hope of recovery ended up there, in their last stages of despair, a prolonged illness having sucked away bodily strength and money. They were treated by an intern and/or a conscientious junior doctor, and the single nurse on duty. Some braved it for a week or two and left, no better for the treatment. Others perished. I don't recall a single patient who benefited from the ordeal of this cruel charity.

The hospital was popular with celebrities, politicians and all those who did not have to worry about money. They came because of some very fine doctors who visited as part-time consultants, this being the norm in big hospitals. What depressed me was the cowardly, deferential attitude of some specialists who must have been aware of the rampant malpractice in the hospital. I talked about it to a few of them. They agreed that all of it was wrong, but preferred to say nothing.

The boss was unhappy with me. I was summoned frequently to his office and admonished for not admitting more patients to the ICU, for not doing enough diagnostic tests, for not making enough money for the hospital; for dressing well. ('Model, eh?' he jibed, during a ward round.) I wonder why I did not fight back harder. Once, he asked me to operate on a patient with haemorrhoids—better known as piles—the term for the tortuous veins stacked at the nether end of our digestive tract. The patient had a serious liver disorder which is a contra-indication for surgery. The liver produces Vitamin K, which is essential for the clotting process and required to seal off small blood vessels damaged during surgery. When I pointed this out, the boss laughed and told me to get on with it. The result was serious post-operative bleeding; after a week of blood transfusions and repeat surgery, the patient succumbed.

I should have refused to do the case, and felt dreadful because there was no way I could have explained it to anyone. The fact remains that the surgeon is responsible.

In the early hours of one Sunday morning, I received an urgent call from the hospital. A young man on a motorbike had collided with a car and sustained grievous injuries to his right arm and leg. There were two fractures in the leg; the arm was crushed at the elbow, damaging the artery and bone. The orthopaedic surgeon offered to fix the bones first so the arterial repair in the arm could be done with the bones in normal position. The Chief, who hated anyone else coming up with a decision, countered him immediately. 'Vascular first,' he cut in. 'We'll send for you as soon as the blood vessels and nerves are repaired and then you fix the bones.' It was a bad decision. The forceful handling of bones, the drilling and fixing of screw and plates after the arterial repair would certainly damage the delicate vascular restoration. I asked the anaesthetist, a very senior man, if he would please speak to the boss. 'He will not listen,' said he, in a low voice and got down to his job of putting the patient to sleep.

I watched in disbelief as the vascular surgeon carried out the delicate procedure of mending the torn artery with a portion of a vein taken from the leg. It was well after noon when the bone specialist began his muscular exertions—pull, press, twist and turn—followed by drilling and nailing to get the broken fragments together. Within minutes, the affronted artery ceased to pulsate. Drugs to revive the collapsed vascular channels and prevent clot-formation did not help. The trauma of the accident compounded by the drama of surgery caused the elbow to swell: closure of the wound became impossible. The boss, who had been walking in and out of the OT through most of the procedure, said, 'Pull. Pull harder! Use heavy sutures!' Nothing doing. The tensile strength of skin and the tissues beneath allowed a fraction of a millimetre of elasticity, not more.

The plastic surgeon was sent for. He came, unhappy to be disturbed on a Sunday evening, and scowled with displeasure on seeing the wound. 'It will need a full-thickness pedicle graft. That must wait until the swelling subsides and the wound is clean.' He advised leaving the wound partially open. As soon as he left, the boss started giving instructions. The wound edges were pulled with greater force and sutured with the thickest material available; the ugly battleground was covered with heavy bandages that extended to cover his entire arm, forearm and the hand. The patient was shifted to the ICU.

Monday morning. I headed for the ICU. When I tried speaking to the patient, he turned away. Anxious, I asked the nurse to undo the bandage which covered the hand. The fingertips were an unhealthy purple, the wrist pulseless, the blood pressure low. Even the antiseptic smells of the ICU could not mask the faint whiff of decay. I called up the anaesthetist (the same who had put him to sleep the previous day). 'The fingers are blue, the radial pulse is absent. It needs a relook, maybe an urgent amputation.' I said. 'I'll arrange for blood…' There were a few seconds of silence before he replied, 'You better wait for the boss.' I started to say that there was a risk of septicaemia, but he hung up.

Outside the ICU, the patient's brother and his young wife were waiting. The boss arrived earlier than usual that day and headed for the ICU. With a sense of urgency, I started to tell him about the poor circulation in the affected arm of the accident victim. His eyes bulged with fury.

'I did not ask for the bandages to be removed,' he thundered. 'How dare you interfere?' He swung round to the nurse. 'Bandage it up properly. Increase the dose of antibiotics…and you—I forbid you to give any orders!'

I should have defended myself. But shocked as I was by his outburst, I was sickened by the fact that not one of the other doctors spoke up for me. It could have been that they had been in similar situations and knew that it was fruitless to argue with the boss.

This tragic performance of 'examining' the sorry limb with the bandages in place went on for two days. Newer antibiotics were added, blood transfused, laboratory tests repeated. By the third day the ICU began to stink of dead flesh and the patient was shifted to a room in a distant corner of a long corridor. Septicaemia led to a drop in blood pressure; his pulse raced and he became disoriented. The family looked on, helpless. On the afternoon of Wednesday the patient was wheeled off to the operating theatre and the arm amputated well above the elbow... He was a twenty-eight-year-old father of two, and drove a mini-van that carted vegetables.

Disasters such as this were more frequent in general-ward patients. Those who could afford private wards were less gullible, and went in search of a better alternative when a patient's progress was suspect. At times an angry patient would threaten to sue the hospital but would be placated with a smaller bill. The surgical catastrophes did not deter the boss who boasted that his five-star hospital was in favour with the then chief minister; indeed, it was. In my capacity as a subordinate to the boss, I was assigned to treat her trusted deputy, the same who had been cooling her heels at the Central Jail in Bangalore till January 2021. I made three visits to the CM's residence to treat a minimally injured big toe (the deputy's) which got knocked against a door-jamb. There were no broken bones but the pain was obviously bad and she asked for a pain-relieving injection. After my first visit, a long, black car would arrive in the afternoon to take me to the CM's residence to check on the patient. (I have clear memory of a stunning photograph of the chief minister in the covered porch of the bungalow, and the heady fragrance of some ghee-drenched delicacy from within.) I will not say that I did not relish being made much of, but on my third visit I had to wait a long while as the lady with the toe was at a meeting. When I did get to see her, I convinced her that she was fit, and stopped my visits.

The summons to the boss's office became frequent. I hated working for the butcherly surgeon who exhibited a gilt-framed portrait of himself in the hospital quadrangle. There were whispers of a psychiatric illness for the treatment of which he made regular trips to the US. But for his efficient and fetching wife who was the administrator, the hospital would have folded up. My ordeal lasted a little over three months at the end of which I went to the office to submit my letter of resignation. The lady said, smiling: 'I'm glad to hear it.' I walked out of the gates and hailed an auto home, consoling myself that this too was a lesson I had to learn.

Thereafter I worked for another year in Madras in circumstances that were vastly better than the one I have recounted. I met several very fine doctors in every field and was not only impressed by their work but inspired, for it is clearly much, much harder to be successful in the true sense in a city than anywhere else. As for me, I liked the independence of being a consulting surgeon in a well-managed hospital. Still I was uncomfortable with certain unwritten rules of city practice. Doctors spent a vast amount of their time speeding from one hospital to the next, meeting the rising demands for specialized care. The best among them were stretched beyond their limits, while others solicited work.* New hospitals drove the once-popular government institutions to the background. Privatized medicine had become popular, but it was also expensive for ordinary people; the quality of nursing was uneven, the rapport

*If you believe in super-busy doctors being the best, hear this: A senior, distinguished surgeon in Madras used to have a night clinic from 9 p.m. to 11 p.m. I asked him why he taxed himself thus. 'Patients think I've had a hectic day till 9 p.m., that I have been operating and saving lives in some other hospital. It's good for my image. What I do is, I stop work at 1 p.m., have a restful afternoon and relax all evening. I come here after an early dinner.'

between doctors and patients, unless cultivated with genuine care, had become a thing of the past. A surgeon in Bombay once told me how he organized his operating lists in four different hospitals. It was a time when laparoscopic surgeries were coming into their own. He was one of the most experienced in the city and in high demand. No sooner had he finished, say, a stomach surgery at one hospital, he would be on his way to tackle a cancerous colon in another hospital 12 kilometres away, even before the first wound had been sutured back in place, much less bandaged and the patient wheeled back to bed. That was left to an assistant. 'My most trusted assistant happens to be my driver,' he said, and seeing my astonishment, explained: 'You don't know what's it's like in this city. It is easy to say, why not a junior doctor. Trouble is, they learn fast and then want to set up practice on their own. But the driver, he is never any competition. And I don't need to pay him as much as I would have to pay a doctor.'

During my tenure of a year and three months in Madras I got paid far more, for far doing little; I earned hundred rupees for every patient I saw as a consultant. Twenty years later, once again in a clinic of my own in Kodagu, my regular consultation fee is Rs 100. There are those who pay Rs 50 or 60 or Rs 150. Ten years ago in a Bombay hospital I paid 800 bucks for five minutes of the doctor's time.

The disparity bothered me; it also made me lazy. I would be home well before Vijay returned from the newspaper office. We had been married three years and were living in Madras when something bit. He talked about quitting his regular job, not because of the job itself but because of his natural inability to work for anyone for too long. He wanted to work from home, and we were both in favour of not going to another city.

15
Change Is Inevitable

We gave up our jobs, bundled up our wealth, boarded the train and two-and-a-half days later, got off at Mokama to be whisked away in the hospital jeep to a warm welcome at the hospital. Thus I made my second sortie into Bihar, for eighteen months, and Vijay wrote his book, *Bihar Is in the Eye of the Beholder* (Viking/Penguin 2000).

Nazareth Hospital had expanded and changed, but not beyond recognition. A new building designed by German architects loomed over the older hospital, appearing a little like an industrial complex, dwarfing all else. With central air-conditioning, the new building was an unsuitable sanctuary for the sick in an impoverished town. You could sense the disappointment among some of the more senior nuns, and murmurs of how the money could have been better spent.

Some gifts, however, cannot be refused.

This upturn also brought several benefits. Better equipment in every department and plenty of space. The work remained as capricious as ever: what more could I ask for? In the nursing school, girls from the north-eastern states now equalled the Malayalis, bringing with them their own cultural richness, like fresh breeze. In Patna, Lalu Prasad Yadav ruled. Having roused the depressed classes to be aware of their entitlements and starting off with great promise, he had begun to falter; serious charges of corruption made him ever more pugnacious and probably too confident. Vijay, who was still contributing to *The Hindu*, took to Mokama with great ease. He returned from one of Lalu's political rallies with vivid descriptions of his ability to charm the crowds. Whatever changes in our political system, this aura around political stars will persist, for a few or several interminable years when the said star can hoodwink millions who are hoodwink-worthy. Government hospitals all over Bihar were without staff, schools were without teachers. Unmanned village health centres and schools were used for cattle.

The Biharis love Bihar. Non-Biharis love it too. Bihar afforded me with personal happiness. Here, violence and folly rub elbows with peace and prudence; wealth and poverty are twins born of the same parent; a gun is an easier buy than a television set; this most confounding of all places is where the Buddha sought enlightenment. My second stint in Bihar was as enriching as the first.

*

The cool interior of a restaurant. On the table before me, a bowl with three scoops of icecream—mango, kesar-pista and rose milk—with a wafer and a cherry on top. In other words, heaven… and then, oh damn!

The cruel shrill summon of the telephone. I got out of bed and picked up the receiver.

'Yes?' I wanted the person at the other end to sense the scowl in my voice, hoping Jayant was the junior doctor on duty and not Arjun. But bad luck, it was Arjun. Jayant was the lazy one and happy enough to hold off any courageous surgery till morning. Not Arjun.*

---

*I was fortunate to have two doctors in the department. Arjun turned out to be an avid learner; he acquired enough skill to do several procedures independently. Jayant too had a good mind but not the inclination to work. Both studied at Patna Medical College, they wrote all their exams in Hindi and

'Perf lag raha hai. Haan, Medum. I think it is a perforation.'

Was he sure? Yes, he was sure. 'They're willing for the surgery,' he added, brightly. 'I've called the OT staff.'

Ten minutes to 12 a.m. I wrapped my sari around my pyjamas, gave my peacefully slumbering husband a murderous look and made my way to the ward. It was perforation all right, in a middle-aged farmer from Baktiarpur. Fortunately, it was a duodenal ulcer and he had been previously quite fit. Just as common were typhoid perforations which are more perilous. Half an hour later we're in green scrubs, bathed in the cold light of the operating lamp. The patient was leanly built, he had been brought to the hospital soon enough, so my task was easier. It was a case I could have taken Arjun through; I knew he's eager to learn. But feeling distinctly crabby about those three scoops of ice cream, I did it myself. He too must get some sleep, his year-old baby had fever he said, and morning's work was barely a few hours away. I finished fast and hurried home, hopeful of sinking back to sleep before the ice cream melted…

'Kavu…I think you'll have to get up.'

I had barely touched the edge of slumber, I was not even properly there.

'Come back here if you know what's good for you,' I said to Vijay. His voice was coming from the sitting room and I knew, even in my drowsy state, that it was hopeless. I opened my eyes to the brightness of the light and to the sight of Vijay taking my white coat off the hook.

'I heard the shots,' he said as I searched for the slippers with my feet. 'It's somewhere close. They'll call you any minute.'

This time, it was Jayant who assisted. Arjun Junior had high fever, so his colleague would take care of the few hours till morning. Jayant was okay for routine cases: varicose veins, an

---

were unable to spell words like hydrocele or cholecystitis. The patient records often had words like 'gabraahat' (fear) 'khujli' (itch) or 'sookhi khansi' (dry cough).

appendix or some simple abdominal surgery. Gunshot wounds are unfailingly fickle, they trick you if you aren't careful. I would have to check everything myself.

At 2.30 a.m., we began operating on the nineteen-year-old known criminal with multiple gunshot wounds to the abdomen, neck and thigh. When we finished, it was Monday morning, cows were being milked, the newspapers had arrived at the station, a motorbike was coming to life somewhere in town, a hospital ayah was opening the door to my outpatient clinic, to sweep and swab.

*

On an another equally grim night I was bent over a belly tattered with multiple shots. I heard behind me a familiar voice conversing in low tones with Bernadette. Mask, cap and the rumpled green theatre garb could not hide the culprit. Vijay was tired of asking me to let him watch a surgery. He had wheedled his way in by charming Bernadette. I'd have to sort him out later, at home. But he managed, and so did the patient, a sub-inspector of police, ambushed by a gang of dacoits hiding inside a sweet shop in town. Bullets had ripped his colon, small intestine and a kidney. He escaped death because the sweet shop was a five-minute drive from the hospital.

*

At times only the most simple intervention, and only that, will come to your rescue. When a policeman trying to intervene between two warring factions took a bullet in his chest, there was no time for any strategy: from the street to the operating table. As alarming as the blood that gushed through wads of dressing pressed over the wound was the way his chest heaved and shuddered, as though hesitating between life and death. This flailing of chest is a sure sign of several fragmented ribs, with bits of bone pressing on the lung, thus impeding the intake of breath. The man submitted without fuss to being lifted off the stretcher onto the operating table, with Sister Margaret shoving a needle into his arm with rougher-than-usual haste. 'He's asleep,' she said, having injected an anaesthetic into his vein. 'You've got to be fast.' Four or five ribs on the left side had broken into multiple bits which flailed helplessly, crushing the lung beneath. Trying furiously to think, I undid the blood-soaked dressing, enlarged the wound with a scalpel and began to scoop out fistfuls of clotted blood from the chest. The patient took infrequent, shuddering breaths of oxygen being fed through a nasal catheter. I could feel the naked heart pressing against my fingers. The shrunken lung cowered beneath palm-sized clots. The simplest solution was to clean out the chest, stick a fat tube-drain into the chest, suture the muscles of the rib-cage and connect the tube to underwater-seal drainage. With all the air that had collected in the chest being drained out, the lung expanded, his breathing became steady; the bleeding seemed to ebb, as though listening to some higher command. Four units of blood, and by morning I knew he had a chance of recovery. Later, speaking to his wife and daughter, I learnt that he was just sixty days short of his retirement.

*

The nuns faced obstacles of every sort: religious, sexist, racist, communal and criminal. No matter how dangerous, they needed to go out of the hospital gates. They went boldly and over the years, established a remarkable rapport with the local people. Compared to the nuns we were timid, walking in the maidan near the chapel after work, chatting with nuns and nurses, visiting the doctors' homes for tea-and-gossip, watching Sunday films with the rest, and star-gazing on clear, clear nights. Nuns, nurses, the pharmacist, shop-owners, hospital cook and other interesting people were part of our social circle. Vijay wheedled his way into the library meant for the Sisters, and was content; he manfully persisted in supervising housework and our part-time maid Pushpa, which meant I did not have to worry about domestic matters.

There was much else about Mokama outside the hospital gates which engrossed Vijay. Once every few months, we escaped to Patna to relish a day of city-life. The nurses went too, very cautiously, in batches. At times a nurse would be alone returning from her visit home to Kerala and that was risky. There were rare instances of intimidation or worse. Vijay went out more often than I did; he made many friends, even whooped it up at a wedding baraat. I had to try and be restrained and sometimes cunning as I had to trod carefully around various types of coercion and threat. Most of them were to do with cases of assault or killing, for which the surgeon has to submit a medical report in court. I was asked to look kindly on the guilty by diluting my report. The favour-seekers would surprise me in the evenings when I walked the short stretch to our flat, or come home to show the earnestness. I was told about the bechara ladka whose reputation would be ruined if he was sent to prison. I listened attentively to the plight of the 'poor boy'. 'Haanji. Phikar mat keejiye. Jo sachch hai, woh hi likhenge.' (Do not fear; I will write only what is true.) It meant that some delectable gifts—fresh river fish, juicy cucumber or tender green lauki—would stop coming. A few months of it and then I was left alone.

*

Inevitably, starting in the 1990s, management culture seeped in. Nuns were sent off to faraway places to learn the art of managing people, besides departments, medicines and money. A degree in hospital administration and management is the coat of arms which apparently improves efficiency. It is corporate philosophy applied to health care. A doctor's job will always be an art and a science, coloured by varying shades of cunning.

Much as I believe in genuine caring as the embodiment of good medical care, every hospital, nursing home or private clinic must aim for financial rectitude *and* self-sufficiency. Professional integrity allows you to accept or refuse charity. Efficiency is essential for balancing expenditure. I am yet to see the steel-cold value system bandied about by hospital administrators and those who head human resource departments teach anyone anything about dealing with people. My experience has yielded nothing but frustration with these well-intentioned men and women.

The hospital in Mokama worked hard to keep abreast of the growing needs of the medical world; it was certainly *managed* very well. But the soul seemed to have gone out of it, just a little. The nuns themselves spoke sadly about disappearing values. About sixty years after its inception, having reflected deeply about the nature of their work and its usefulness to society, the nuns concluded that they must change course. They decided to concentrate on preventive health care and alternate medicine. It was by no means easy to shut down the wards, which meant that they would have to retrench hundreds of employees who had built their careers and their lives at the hospital. Now, I am told, the hospital is open for outpatient care, alternate medical care, the treatment of chronic diseases like tuberculosis and leprosy, the treatment of HIV/AIDS, geriatric care and the training of community health workers. To accept change and to rearrange your methods to suit the needs of that region is smart thinking.

16

A Hol(e)y Health Care

'We have left undone things we ought to have done; and we have done things we ought not to have done; and there is no health in us.'—The Book of Common Prayer

I found that I had been abraded by the rough and tumble of Uttar Pradesh and Bihar. Much as I loved the work and the people, I grew tired of treating injured dacoits in the night. Besides, the doctor who treats is not allowed a single yellowed bullet as a keepsake. Violent injuries are medico-legal. The bullet has to be submitted in court via the police, along with a detailed report of the injury, the treatment and outcome. The vengeful summers and bitter winters, the erratic hours of work and a nostalgia for the effete tranquillity of the south began to tell on our resilience.

A friend informed us of a sixty-bed hospital in Idukki district of Kerala run by a senior doctor, who was a Licentiate Medical Practitioner (LMP).* So we bid a tearful goodbye to

*In pre-independent India, this shorter medical course enabled one to obtain the certificate of an LMP and practice as a doctor. When the number of medical colleges offering the full-fledged medical course of MBBS increased, the LMP courses were stopped, and these early practitioners were allowed to complete the MBBS degree if they wished.

everything and everyone that we had held dear in Mokama and boarded the train that would take us to another Promised Land, all of three days' journey away.

Kerala, known the world over as a narrow strip of coastal splendour, never fails to surprise. Their common language of Malayalam is a unifying strength. Them 'mallus' are everywhere; they evoke a mix of envy and ire because of their genius for prosperity as trader, trickster, pujari, poet, jeweller, artist, scholar and saint. The land of Adi Shankara (who abrogated the caste system as early 8th century CE) is also where exorcists, shamans and modern-day charlatans thrive. And yet, in Kerala it does not matter if you eat a certain type of meat or pray to a deity or believe in miracles or wear a skull-cap or swear loyalty to a godhead supposedly from Europe. Sadly, this everyday harmony of life is set to change.

Vijay's ancestral home is in the small village of Thayyur near Yermapetty in Kerala's Thrissur district. I am in awe of the restrained lifestyle of the Nambisans and the unique flavour of their culture. But that was a good distance away from Idukki where I had accepted the job. The privately owned hospital belonged to Dr T. He was a soft-spoken, genial bear of a man in his late seventies; he was hard-working and earnest in his efforts. There were two other doctors—one with a diploma in anaesthesia and the other with a diploma in paediatrics.

The very first day at work I felt a churn of doubt and disappointment with the slapdash, hit-or-miss nature of ward routine. The nursing care, ward cleanliness, the laboratory and surgical facilities were poor; the doctors came and went at different times; patients and attendants flocked in at all hours. The hospital waste was chucked right behind the operating theatre, which was itself shabby. The staff had no concept of asepsis.

Each day began with a prayer aired through a loudspeaker. Patients enfeebled by illness and meek religious faith trailed in, with folded hands; they bowed to the doctor who blessed them chastely, with a hand over their heads. I begged off this uncomfortably pretentious morning assembly after a couple of days.

Dr T saw all types of patients and performed surgeries. He was adored, the way some religious people are. When I complained to him about the serious drawbacks in the hospital, he evinced genuine concern and a desire to improve things. He said he had been helpless to do anything single-handed. Together, we chalked out a plan. With a dozen potential nurse trainees, I began to take classes. A routine was put in place for ward-hygiene and surgical asepsis. I went with Dr T to Kochi (Kozhikode) to buy an autoclave, surgical instruments, linen for the nurses' uniforms, sheets, blankets, toilet essentials, dozens of buckets in graded sizes, rat and cockroach exterminators and gallons of phenyl. I became obsessed with the task set out for me and worked in earnest.

What was I expecting? I sensed the first sign of disgruntlement from the anaesthetist. Vijay and I had dropped in at his living quarters and we were having tea. 'You will either fit in here, or you won't,' he told me, bluntly. 'You join a hospital, be willing to accept its norms. Don't go chasing after some dream which matters to no one else.' I got into an argument with him. When we got up to leave, the doctor just sat there, his lips tight and stubborn.

The paediatrician was genuinely concerned about all that was wrong in the hospital and readily agreed to help. It took several weeks to get the nurses and ayahs to adjust, for they too were accustomed to being casual. Eventually matters began to improve. I was pleased. The eagerness of the new trainee nurses gave me hope. I went to the boss every day with a list of things to be bought, rules to be made compulsory, problems to be solved. He listened to me with an uncommunicative smile on his benign face and invariably ended the session by inviting us to dinner at his home. He was a widower, living with his son and daughter-in-law. The food was wonderful.

Over time, I realized that he had not, for a moment, shared my beliefs or thought my efforts to change anything in the hospital were worthwhile. It was *his* hospital and I was a salaried employee. After spending a lakh or so on the improvements, he became indifferent. He talked to me about doing more surgery but for all the wrong reasons. Half the number of pregnant women who came to the hospital ended up with a Caesarean Section to have the baby. I refused to do them if the decision was not mine. We argued and finally he gave in, saying, I could decide how I handled my patients and he would decide about his.

One day while operating, I heard the door open and someone walk in. I looked up to find Dr T's son, an uncouth, lumbering giant of a man. I had heard rumours about his conduct with the nurses, and his wife had once complained to me about his philandering ways. He stood at the entry to the operating room in his street clothes and sandalled feet, rubbing his stomach; grinning. 'I just came to see you operate,' he said. 'I want to watch.'

The scene that followed ended with me losing my carefully controlled temper and telling him to get out. Dr T later tried to reassure me. 'He does not mean any harm.'

My work suffered for several days afterwards. Checking some medicines one afternoon, I found that expired drugs were being sold at the hospital pharmacy. I questioned the pharmacist.

'No problem,' he said coolly. 'Who checks these things?'

He assured me that he would henceforth snip off the dates on the tablet strips. This time when I complained to Dr T, he did not smile. 'If you don't like it here, it is better to leave,' he said, softly.

What is one to do in such a situation? In a few days, the

decision was made for me. I received a letter in a pink envelope: my marching orders. It was our wedding anniversary. We lunched at the best of the affordable restaurants in the area, defiantly blowing up our precious funds and surveyed our future. I had lasted a mere five months at the job.

By definition, a rolling stone is positioned on an incline. Roll you will, but if you stay centred inside yourself, it is a little bit easy. You might gather more bruises than moss, which is all right if you remember that a moment will arrive when you must stay tenaciously put.

17
The Rural Hospital

May I take a short diversion before getting back to my story?

The bumpiness of a medical ride in India is all too familiar. The faith that society places on doctors helps to make us what we are. It is essential that we evolve and re-form within the framework of society. Doctors thrive on the feeling of *usefulness*, as much as the scope that work offers for our own betterment. Rural practice suits me well. This chapter is the sketch of a hospital apposite to such work, the intention being to be able to treat a wide range of cases at a cost that does not pinch an average citizen. The ideal hospital is a frequently argued topic at the annual conclave of surgeons like myself who work in far-flung places in various parts of our country and the world. My views here include much of this received wisdom.

The last decade of my surgical career was at a rural hospital in Kodagu, Karnataka. I began life in Kodagu and it would be fitting if I could finish my final years in this very place. My 'pyare watan'. My ideal of a rural hospital has much in common with the one I worked at, and which goes by the simple name of Rural India Health Project Hospital. Very government-sounding. But no, it is a hospital that was started by a few committed local people in the 1960s.

Half an acre of land, in the heart of a town or village will suffice for a twenty- or thirty-bedded hospital. Compactness means fewer staff, better team-work and a higher degree of satisfaction. The wards, the delivery room, operating theatre and the ancillary departments must be within easy reach of doctors and nurses, or they will spend time and energy in wheeling trolleys and stretchers through long corridors or negotiating them in and out of lifts and sparing patients, weakened by age and illness, the discomfort of being trundled about.

In hospitals of elephantine dimensions, doctors rely on reports pasted into the patients' records or see them on the computer screen. There is very little scope for doctors to meet and exchange views.

In large hospitals, many surgeons are occupied in as many theatres. The scene is much like that in an anthill, with unceasing, repetitive activity. Once in a while an ant misses a step and in the split-second it takes to steady itself, the damage is done. In the midst of the hurry and worry that are a part of sickness, medical mishaps occur, more often due to carelessness than due to neglect or incompetence. Does anyone recall the instance of the mother of a well-known Indian actress being operated on the wrong side of the brain for a tumour? It was in the 1990s at a leading centre in the US. The X-rays shown to the surgeon in the operating room belonged to another patient whose tumour was on the opposite side. If the surgeon, focused on the details of the procedure, is working on a semi-automatic gear setting, s/he will not stop to think, 'Which patient is this?' but will rely on the X-rays put up by a theatre assistant, which may result in unforgivable errors.

My mother was in her seventies when she was advised surgery for a thyroid swelling. It was at one of the best hospitals in Delhi. On the morning of the surgery, she was woken early, given the shapeless hospital gown to change into and her hair tucked into a cap; the ear and nose rings were removed, wrapped in a handkerchief and handed over to us; her pulse and blood pressure were recorded. She climbed on to a hospital trolley and was wheeled away to the operating theatre, with her two anxious daughters following. At the entrance to the operating complex, two nurses in green scrubs and masks shifted her onto the operating-room stretcher and wheeled her in. By this time, my mother, well under the influence of the preoperative sedative, was dozing peacefully.

Just as the stretcher was being moved into the operating theatre, I heard one of the nurses say, 'She's the gall bladder, for OT 3.'

'No, she isn't!' I cried. 'She's the thyroid!'

The mistake would have been discovered when the anaesthetist checked the case records. But what if the anaesthetist had also got mixed up and my sleeping mother had had her gall bladder removed instead of the thyroid?

Serious illness can make us lose control over our independence, our sense of dignity and life. It is a tremendous loss and a personal one. Hospital is where we end up when illness leaves us with no other choice. The ordeal of medicines, injections, laboratory tests, well-intentioned nurse-intrusions and the perpetual, mostly depressing sounds have to be borne during a hospital stay. Artificially lit windowless enclosures filled with the hospital sundry of drip stands, oxygen cylinders, suction pumps and bed-rails with which a patient can be fenced in, are not exactly pleasing. Smaller hospitals have many advantages, like the two health-giving freebies: sunlight and fresh breeze. Cheery, well-ventilated wards help the patients in their recovery, and enable the staff to work in comfort. The practice of having windows and then sealing them off (and curtaining them for good measure) in order to install air conditioners is ridiculous. Air conditioning does not guarantee clean interiors, and is useful only in extreme weather conditions. Unless scrupulously maintained, it causes more harm than good. In most parts of our country, air conditioning is not required while in others it is necessary during the hot summer months.

If the supply of electricity is erratic as in most small towns and all of rural India, it is impossible to use air conditioners without good generator backup.

The facilities provided in the general wards are basic and should therefore be thoughtfully planned: a distance of six feet between the beds, a locker for each person and where possible, curtains between the beds is ideal. Indian-style toilets are easier to keep clean. For recently operated patients and for those with stiff joints, a wooden seating arrangement which is placed over the toilet can be made by a local carpenter.

Critical, life-threatening cases land up in the emergency ward and therefore it must be equipped with oxygen, anaesthesia and suctioning machines, nebulizers, cardiac monitors and urgent, life-saving medicines. Emergencies are capricious. You confront tragedy, horror, cruelty, violence and madness at unexpected moments. What words of comfort to offer the man whose wife has sliced off his penis for adultery? How do you console a mother whose mentally disturbed daughter of thirteen is seven months pregnant? What does the doctor tell the unreformed alcoholic and two-time divorcee who swears he loves her and no one else? Or the fifty-year-old who survived a suicide attempt a quarter of a century ago but was paralyzed for life by a bullet and is brought by his older brother in a wheelchair every month for a change of tubes that drain his bladder? Life is as colourful as it is grim.

I have been assaulted by a drug addict, threatened by criminals, solicited by drunks, abused by idiots who think they have the right to exclusive treatment, belittled, abused, flattered and offered genuine gratitude. The occasional moments of mirth more than make up for the darker moments. One of the best scenes (for the rest of my team, not me) was when a grateful patient rushed at me as we were coming out of the male ward and fell at my feet, with effusive thankfulness for treating his mother. Embarrassed, I tried to stop him; he rose abruptly, colliding against my chin. I was dizzy for a moment but managed to regain my composure and proceeded on rounds, trying to rub away the soreness with as much dignity as I could. I was well aware of the mirth that followed me. By the time I reached home the lower half of my face was streaked with a dusky blue ink-splash of a bruise. I had to manage with that for an entire week while team-mates chuckled, with caution. At home, Vijay did it openly.

The operating theatre is positioned well away from the wards and closed off from the rest of the hospital by swing doors and the NO-ENTRY sign. It includes the sterilization wing where surgical instruments and linen are sterilized, cubicles for the change of clothes, a sitting area for doctors and nurses and a toilet. Here too, one can source freebies, up to a point. Sunlight is allowed to stream in through large, minimally tinted glass-paned windows. It is often enough for minor procedures. When electricity fails one can safely continue with the help of a big torch and use a foot-operated suction machine until the standby generator kicks in. The windows are not opened except when the theatre is being cleaned, and exhaust fans are used to allow fresh air to circulate. The hospital in Kodagu, where I work, was planned and designed by some very fine minds. It is a tile-roofed building with large deep windows and airy wards. The operating theatre is well lit by natural light. There is nothing as soothing as the view of a tree-lined garden while you scrub and gown for surgery.

A lot of hospital activity orbits round the operating theatre and the Intensive Care Unit (ICU). Rules regarding entry and exit, change of footwear and clothing are absolute. And not to be compromised. I once saw a senior, much respected gynaecologist in a major hospital operating with her long plait dangling from behind the sterile cap on her head. There are surgeons who make a habit of walking in and out of the operating complex in scrubs, mask and cap, in a showy gesture of importance and haste. Microorganisms disregard such misconduct, and will strike back with an infection in the just-operated patient. When called to attend to a dire emergency outside the operating theatre, if the surgeon does rush out in surgical scrubs, he must change into a fresh sterile set on re-entry.

Simple surgeries, dressings and fracture reductions are done in a minor operating room. Some hospitals have what is called a 'septic theatre', meaning the little side-room where you lance boils, drain abscesses and dress maggot-ridden wounds.

The ICU is for critically ill patients who need constant care and monitoring of their vital functions like the heartbeat, breathing, the status of consciousness and urine output. Some need it for a few days; others, for a longer period. ICU work is very, very specialized. It demands a thorough knowledge of the many vital functions of the body which keep one alive. It is a facility which demands complex equipment, specially trained staff and round-the-clock vigilance. It is also a place where, more than anywhere else, one must not let go of common sense. That may sound paradoxical: patients in an ICU are critically ill; their body dynamics are fragile and may change in seconds. The doctors and nurses need to be constantly vigilant, and while utilizing the critical-care gadgets effectively, must not lose sight of the most obvious: a patient is a whole, living entity and not a mere collection of organs and systems to be repaired. The ICU staff need to maintain equanimity when talking to relatives who are anxious about the outcome of the illness, and worried about the mounting expenses. ICU facilities come at an exorbitant cost; wasteful expenditure is always wrong.

The conditions in rural environments being different, an ICU is best managed when it is small and adequately equipped. One spacious, well-ventilated room with three or four beds will suffice. The cardiac monitor, defibrillator, pulse oxymeter and a ready supply of oxygen are the first essentials. (Centrally piped oxygen is still a luxury and one can do well enough with oxygen cylinders, the supply of which has improved in recent years.) After watching a few specialized centres in multi-speciality hospitals, I am certain that ICU procedures can be taught to those who work in rural areas by deputing them to a higher centre for a short period and thereafter, encouraging them to learn at work.

Next comes the pharmacy, which consists of a main store where the drugs are tabulated and stocked. And a smaller dispensing outlet from where medicines are purchased as required by the patients. Even a small hospital stocks hundreds of items which include life-saving drugs, anti-snakebite and anti-rabies serum, vaccines and a carefully selected range of antibiotics. If and when higher antibiotics are needed, they can be procured in eight to twelve hours, from a stockist in the city who will send it by the next bus. This should be standard practice and not mere frugality, as a precaution against antibiotic overuse. Drug resistance* is already rampant. It is the curse of many city hospitals, particularly in India where over-the-counter sale of drugs is common and uncontrolled.

X-ray, ultrasound and a properly equipped laboratory make up the other departments. The skill and aptitude of those who conduct the tests is as important as the quality of the testing devises. It is far better to be reliable in doing the most commonly required laboratory tests (there are about two dozen of these) than to be lavish and unreliable. Rural hospitals struggle to maintain good laboratories.

Our district, with a population just under 6 lakh, has had to manage with a single blood bank which is 70 kilometres away from the hospital where I work.

*The indiscriminate use and overuse of an antibiotic results in the microbes developing defence mechanisms against the drug, thus rendering them useless in treating infections. Medical expertise predicts that the next great pandemic will be from microbes which become resistant to antibiotics, antivirals, antifungals and anti-parasitic drugs.

Procuring blood thus takes too much time and effort, and in urgent cases, defeats the purpose. Rural hospitals around the country have practised another method for decades. It is called Unbanked Direct Blood Transfusion or UDBT—which is to take the blood directly from a healthy individual (usually a relative) and transfuse it, after doing the mandatory tests as specified by the WHO. I have done so through my entire rural career without problems. Even minor side-effects like fever, rash and joint pains are uncommon and short-lived. As per our laws, this procedure of using fresh compatible blood that has been properly tested for safety is illegal, and permitted only 'in cases where the lack of blood poses a grave risk to life'. 'As during a war,' the law states. In what way will law help a pregnant woman bleeding furiously into her belly, or a young boy who has fallen off a tree and ruptured his spleen, or a young man who has suffered grievous injury in a major road accident? Not to speak of all those others who are so anaemic they must have blood during or soon after surgery and don't have the means to procure it from faraway blood banks?* Health officials from the district headquarters question rural doctors about UDBT and warn about the possible closure of the hospital. Like dozens of rural practitioners everywhere, I explain my reasons for breaking the law and carry on, firm in the belief that rural lives are as precious as those of battling soldiers. UDBT is safe as long as the fundamental rules of blood transfusion are strictly followed.†

---

*A rough calculation: If I have used direct fresh blood transfusions say 5000 times in my entire career, there are at least another thousand surgeons like me with similar numbers. That is 50 lakh patients whose need for blood was fulfilled by using this simple method. If we had all obeyed the dictates of a law that has not thought through the reality of rural surgical work, what would have happened to these lives?

†Surgeons in Orissa and Bengal faced legal action, resulting in a drastic reduction in the number of surgeries. We can only guess how long it will take for blood banks to be within reach for every hospital (all-day and all-night

The buying of equipment for a hospital eats up money. To imitate our sister-hospitals in the cities where specialist-doctors need technology-driven services is unsound. The rural community is largely poor and lower middle class and we owe them medical expertise at prices that are affordable. One has to match need with quality, durability and serviceability. Expensive equipment often lies unused in many government hospitals because the staff has not been trained in its use or it has broken down and no one thought to secure a maintenance contract.

Hospitals evolve; they must. A luxury today might become an essential a few years hence. But it makes no sense to buy equipment that you are likely to use only a few times in a year. In the Kodagu hospital we had a ventilator which is a life-saving equipment but only useful if there is a doctor trained in its use. I think we used it only six or seven times in three years for patients with respiratory failure who could then be shifted to a higher centre. It was an expensive gadget that we could barely afford.

A hygienic kitchen providing wholesome food is an obvious need. Wood and charcoal are best done away with and if in use, a proper chimney or chute should be in place. Steam-cooking, though initially expensive, is probably the best way of maintaining cleanliness and quality. A kitchen garden with seasonal vegetables is a great idea for procuring fresh vegetables, while composted kitchen waste makes organic manure.

The waste produced by a hospital consists of body parts, soiled dressings, contaminated syringes, needles, gloves, plastic tubings and bags, besides food waste. It carries a high risk of spreading disease. The indifference of municipalities and

---

availability of electricity must come before that) but till then? The three-and-a-half litres of the red life fluid racing inside me starts to heat up when I think of the hundreds and thousands of lives that will be lost because of this fundamental shortcoming.

hospitals towards waste is terrifying. The method we found useful was to ensure that waste is collected in separate colour-coded bins; the infected, biodegradable material such as soiled dressings, bandages, the placenta and other excised parts are burnt in an incinerator; plastics and syringes are best collected at a recycling unit where they can be cleaned, sterilized, shredded and reused. This is rarely possible in rural areas and the cost of transporting the material to such a facility in a city is expensive. The next best method is to empty them into a large, deep cement-lined pit. If the plastic is weighted down with soil sprinkled once a week, the pit can accommodate the plastics for many years without contaminating ground water; needles are treated with hypochlorite solution and buried. When complete and safe disposal of bio-hazardous waste is accepted as a priority, we can stop creating these cemeteries for the disease-carrying material that hospitals turn out every day.

Living quarters for hospital staff are best provided near or within the hospital campus. I have had this advantage through most of my working life. It feels good to step out of your home and be at work in a few minutes, and to be home as soon as you are finished. If you are a junior, having the senior doctor close at hand to deal with serious emergencies is a real advantage.

The success or failure of a hospital rests ultimately with the doctors, nurses and other staff. We sometimes overlook the facility of reaching out to the patient, thereby making them feel ignored or rebuffed. To touch and to talk to every patient is the simplest way of caring; it is also the most ignored. *The hospital exists for the patients.* If a patient is dissatisfied, the hospital must address the problem and involve the staff concerned, in the process.

Ward rounds are meant for checking the progress or decline of patients, and making course-corrections. Well-constructed ward rounds improve the quality of care and act as a binding force between the medical team and the patient. But if you want to do the rounds right, you had better be willing to take the time to acknowledge each human being whether patient or team member. The senior-most doctor regulates the rounds, and must do this without making it officious or harsh, and without the loud censure of juniors or nurses. Ward rounds are always about treating the patient and learning from each case. Each problem should be discussed, and choice of treatment decided.

They can also have their lighter moments. Inevitably, the personality and nature of the boss colours the rounds and if s/he is the dour sort, there may be no lighter moments but that is rare. If there is a joke, it is best to share it with the patient or if it is not appropriate, reserve it for later.* I cannot stress this strongly enough. The way we behave with our patients is of crucial importance. What is breezily referred to as 'bedside manners' is nothing but genuine concern towards the sick, without which of what use our knowledge and expertise? Sadly, in the Indian context, rudeness from 'authority' is tolerated without question. Ill-mannered doctors are an extension of society.

A rural hospital must deal with the medico-legal aspects of cases that are criminal in nature, or appear suspicious. Suicide attempts, burns, road accidents, assaults, stabbings and gunshot wounds all fall under the rubric of the medico-legal. The medical findings given in a doctor's report will be used by the police in investigating the cause, and followed up in court. There will, at times, be pressure on the hospital staff to falsify records or deviate from the actual findings to suit someone. Coercion and bribes might come in the way of professional conduct. All it takes is firmness. Such requests eventually stop, along with the offer of money, holiday bargains, air tickets or fresh fish.

---

*Once, at the bedside of an aged man the boss said, in all courtesy: 'Mr B…I have to put my finger in your back passage…I hope you don't mind?'

'Oh that's all right, doc,' came the quick reply. 'Just be sure you don't leave it behind.'

It is necessary to be on good terms with the local police. If treated with courtesy, they will return the compliment. A few cases require the doctor's presence in court, which is all right if there is consideration for the doctor's time. When summons are issued for appearance in court and postponed on the day of hearing, it seriously upsets hospital routine. At other times, I have waited the entire day, sitting on a bench outside the court, waiting to give my report. Most private hospitals refuse to take medico-legal cases because of such inconvenience. In contrast, the court appearances of doctors in court in the UK were pleasing: a police officer would escort the doctor to court, offer tea during the wait, which was never for more than half an hour. The law-makers were precise as well as courteous; when the statement had been made and questions answered, the doctor was escorted back.

A hospital can reach out to the community in different ways. One-day workshops on nutrition, infant care, yoga, waste disposal or stress reduction work extremely well and can be held regularly. A hospital suited to local needs is the true face of health care.

18

Corporate Medical Wisdom

There was no avoiding the consequences of the pink envelope which reached my hands after five months in Idukki. I tried to put up a fight by writing a registered letter to the Medical Council of India (MCI). Vijay and I would trudge two kilometres to the post office every afternoon, sure that there would be a reply. There was none.

We were urgently in need of sustenance, that is, we had to have at least one salaried job between us. With Vijay at the wheel of our agreeably aged and sparingly used Mahindra jeep, we toured the length and breadth of Idukki district in search of a hospital that would want me. I was confident of my worth and so for weeks we knocked about dusty roads in the district and beyond, showing up at many hospitals. I appeared before a few interview committees and spoke truthfully about my last job (foolishly, I realize now), including the letter to the MCI. I was politely turned away. Trouble-making Lady Doctor! No job wanted me. That is a clear and definite, never-to-be-forgotten sensation, with the clarity of a toothache.

Two months went by. The tenancy of our home would expire in a few weeks. We had a hired television and time in excess. Vijay the freelancer had the enviable ability to minimize work and I had no work. We treated ourselves to a happy number of Tamil, Malayalam and Hindi films; we watched cricket, football, tennis, golf, snooker and the Grand Prix. I became a fan of all sport. My cheering would have annoyed some, since I have a tendency to side with the team which seems more worthy of victory, whichever state or country it may represent.

Life however is not all sport and there were tasks to be fulfilled. I...cooked. Cooking for two hungry people is manageable, and housekeeping is dead easy, if you have the knack of kicking things out of the way. (If it is anything delicate, you push.) We stayed for a few soothing weeks in Vijay's ancestral home in the village of Erumapatty in Thrissur and then with a cousin in Kochi where, in the evenings, Vijay and he talked communism over whisky shots. An excellent time was had by all.

On hearing that the poet Kamala Das lived in the city and having met her previously in Madras, we chanced a visit. It is easy to understand why Kamala was so loved by all who knew her. She had a childlike curiosity about everyone and everything. Over freshly fried sweet appams, banana chips and tea we gossiped, the way writers do. When she heard about my non-existent job, Kamala was concerned. Vijay and I had just enough between us to smile bravely, and she understood. 'Give me a minute. I need to make a call,' she said, vanishing into her room. Moments later she was back. 'I spoke to a friend. There is a Tata Tea Hospital in Munnar, and they are in need of a surgeon. You should apply.'

Thus I nosed in, with some eagerness, into the corporate world as surgeon at a hospital in Munnar. The new-found comforts and the courtesy extended by the company were very pleasing. To work in a well-managed hospital was a relief. The etiquette, methods and many niceties of 'Plantation-Culture', however, took getting used to. Eight months later I was transferred to their hospital in the Anamallais (the elephant hills in Tamil Nadu) where the medical department was smaller, and I was in charge.

Anamallai is wild country. The Tata Tea plantations are spread over hilly terrain that lies within the embrace of a wildlife sanctuary. Deer, porcupine, rabbit and peacock visited our garden, blue-flecked whistling thrush sang riotous melodies, rust-winged chembookas belted out their song and moths the size of hand-held fans pressed against the window panes asking to come in; elephants trampled through surrounding land in search of water, leopards coughed within earshot, bisons and wild dogs were sighted after dark; snakes of every hue and potency were commonplace. The high point of our first few months in Anamallai was the hair-clip made out of porcupine quills that Vijay gifted me on my birthday. The spiny creatures roamed freely in our garden, gnawing away our vegetable patch and shedding bits of their armour. Once, a jackfruit kept to ripen in the kitchen emboldened a porcupine to chew away a several inches of our backdoor, leaving behind a gift of varnish-brown quills. The door had to be reinforced with an underskirt of metal sheeting, and I got a designer hair-clip that no amount of money can buy.

*

The Uralikal Central Hospital functioned in such a setting, with four doctors, six nurses and two ward boys. We worked under the protective umbrella of the company. Surprises, however, were never far away.

Four-year-old Pavana had insisted on going with his father to the shop not half a kilometre away to buy jaggery and coconut. It was Pongal the next day and his mother did not want to run out of these essentials. Pavana was dressed in a shirt that hung low enough to hide modesty, the shirt being a suitable apparel in families with more children than they pray for. Clothes must last through several kids. The shatte (Tamil for shirt) serves as a single piece of clothing. When young boys want to pee there are no impedimenta like buttons and zips.

Pavana's father held his little hand as they walked. Caution is ingrained in every adult in Uralikal and the other villages that flourish quietly in the foothills of the Anamallais. Come dusk and no child is seen outside the hutments, so real is the danger of a four-footed predator that hunts for anything smaller than itself. The lush vegetation is home to many a wild beast, particularly the leopard.

There was half an hour to sundown. Father and son sang as they walked and did not hear any sound behind them, until it was too late.

At the hospital gates 40 kilometres away, darkness had wrapped itself around the teashop where Velu was brewing a kettle of tea when the jeep swerved into view. A man peered out. 'Hospital?' Velu nodded, pointing the way and the jeep sped, raising a cloud of dust. Adjacent to the hospital in the surgeon's home, the doctors had gathered with their families for a relaxed Saturday evening. The smell of parippuvadais and coffee wafted from the kitchen. The emergency call came just as they were being served. End of party. Beginning of a nightmare.

Pavana had been attacked by a leopard and had been driven 40 kilometres through gutted roads. He had a single deep wound beneath the rib cage through which a loop of bowel protruded, like an angry tongue. Two jagged tears in his small intestine and a ruptured blood vessel. The damaged portion of the bowel was removed and he was transfused fresh blood from his father. Pavana healed well and went home after fourteen days. The family was able to pay eight hundred rupees before the surgery and the remaining amount when he left.

The British started coffee- and tea-growing in India (Assam, south-west Karnataka and in the hilly tracts of Kerala and Tamil Nadu), as also in parts of Ceylon and Burma in the mid-19th century. Large swathes of forest land were cleared for this new enterprise. A few decades earlier, the Act for the abolishment of slave trade had been passed by the British Parliament. It made slavery punishable by law within the British Empire. Now who was to work in their sugar plantations in Africa and in the coffee and tea plantations of the Asian subcontinent? So almost simultaneously they introduced the system of indentured labour whereby contractors were permitted to bring workers in large numbers under a contract of thus-many years for a specified salary. With this, the British cunningly protected themselves from being shot in the foot. Thousands of indentured labourers sent to the African continent chose to stay on, went into small-time trade and ensured secure futures for their future generations. In India, for nearly a century while the plantations flourished, the workers lived in abominable hardship and poverty. In *Red Tea*, a novel by Paul Harris Daniel, an Indian doctor who worked in one of the plantations of Anamallais tells the brutal story of the cruelty inflicted on illiterate and timid folk desperate for livelihood. In the tea gardens of India, their living conditions were shabby and unsafe. There was violence and deprivation. Once employed, the workers could not leave the area even if they wished, because they were paid in coins minted for use only in a few local shops.

It had to end and it did, well before India wrested freedom from the British. Rules were put in place to ensure the welfare of workers. Prevention of disease and cure were stressed upon in the Plantation Act which came into force in the years following Independence. The labour unions fighting for the rights of manual workers became more active, and succeeded in getting a better deal for the labour force.

Private companies like the Tatas, Hindustan Lever, Parry Agro, British Burma Trading Corporation and dozens of others maintain their own plantation hospitals and dispensaries. Immunizations, mother and child welfare, nutrition, safe drinking water, sanitation and garbage disposal are part of the welfare measures. A crèche where mothers can leave their young children when they go to work is a mandatory requirement in large estates. Regular inspections and medical audits are carried out and shortcomings are addressed consistently, making company-owned plantations one of the fairest employment sectors for a daily-wage earner.

An overhead view of an estate will show the tea gardens as neatly bald patches of light green with clumps of forestland in between. The six estates managed by the Tata group covered a radius of 50 kilometres, with the hospital as its medical hub. Patients like the boy Pavana were non-company. We could have treated many more such serious cases if the hospital was closer to one of the small, populous towns adjoining the plantations. With its location inside the forest area, and given the dreadful state of the roads and the lack of regular bus service, villagers found it difficult to use its facilities more often.

Well-managed plantations facilitate the upward mobility of workers and their families. Schooling allowance for children, scholarships and prizes for outstanding students have ensured that every child goes to school and many to college. A few have become engineers, bankers, doctors, nurses. Professor Thangavelu, who taught at Madras University for a number of years before he became one of the medical advisors for Tata Plantations, was the son of a labourer from the Anamallais. I met him in his sunset years during a medical audit which includes the inspection of the homes of workers. Thangavelu would tell them to keep windows open and let fresh breeze ventilate their homes. 'We used to shut the windows, believing that disease was carried into homes by cold draughts of wind,' he said. 'We did not know that fresh air is essential for keeping off germs.'

At the Uralikal hospital we tried to manage all varieties of cases and only a small number were referred to hospitals in Coimbatore for medical or surgical expertise that we did not possess. The four-hour drive in an ambulance over the hill roads with forty-eight hairpin bends was best avoided. We took care of ruptured pregnancies, twisted guts, broken limbs as well as non-surgical emergencies like heart attacks, snake bites, diabetic coma and stroke. I liked working for the plantations because they cared about the welfare of its workers. It came with a good salary, a bungalow and perks!

My administrative duties turned out to be more demanding than the surgery. Prior to this job, as a doctor, the office was where I went to submit leave applications, collect salary slips, or to meet the administrator if some problem needed her attention. There would be a polite, unyieldingly stern secretary at the typewriter or computer. I would walk in, get my work done and walk out. Now I had an office of my own where I sat for a few hours every day signing registers, approving or declining leave applications, taking note of complaints, meeting union leaders. I frequently went for meetings at the head office, 10 kilometres away. These head-office meetings took half a day. They were not difficult, but taxing. I tax easily.

Bigger meetings were held in Munnar. My job entailed several trips a year for this reason. A five-hour drive through the Muddumalai wildlife sanctuary (deer, wild-boar, jackal, bison and elephant sighted every time) and an overnight stay at the classy High Range Club are not to be scoffed at. The clubs in the plantations are where you see the dying embers of British nostalgia glowing a warm orange and where we, the desi men and women, take on a distinctive sheen. The bar is well stocked and cheap, the 'Marys' are bloody fabulous. At times Vijay came along with me, and we had the time of our lives. The meetings, however, were largely un-inspiring. This was my fault entirely, because all of it should have been a learning experience.

The conference hall was courtly in size, the chairs were comfortably padded and the long table had room enough for forty-eight elbows. Managers, senior managers, unit-heads and a few sub-unit heads like me were present. I sat with over fifteen or twenty smartly turned-out gentlemen and the head of the research department who was a lady and listened to the nuances of tea-growing, picking, curing and processing. I counted bald heads, the spectacled, the big-bellied and the trim; I wondered which of the men would come to hospital with a niggling pain that might be cardiac. I thought about lunch. Medical matters came up in the last ten minutes of the meeting, maybe twenty. I had my moment, and then it would be time for lunch.

Why are plantation employees, at the management level, almost exclusively male? The jobs involve a fair bit of trudging up craggy, sloping pathways and bumping and bounding about in jeeps; and so perhaps is more suited for men. But women in large numbers are hard at work in the fields and there is a fair sprinkling of us among doctors, and also in the staff grade, working as typists and personal assistants. Management work in plantations is demanding. It certainly demands a love of the outdoor life, but it is not physically or intellectually arduous. The 'xy' puzzle remains unsolved.

All plantation groups have three categories of employees: Labourers, Staff and Managers. The divisions are clear and inflexible, the demarcating lines drawn thick and black. At times it was puzzling. A few weeks after I joined work in Munnar, I invited one of the nurses who happened to live close to our living quarters home for tea. The manager of the estate where our house was situated dropped by soon after.

'Kavery, it's not done,' he said. 'You're her boss, and in charge of the hospital.'

'I'm her boss at work.'

He gave me a measured smile. 'We're management grade, the nurses are staff. We don't mix socially.' The nurse too had been told off.

Managerial exclusivity sometimes becomes arrogance, and occasionally dips embarrassingly low. An assistant manager who used to visit us at home told us about a colleague of his who insisted on switching on every light in his bungalow as soon as he returned from work, because it made him feel good. He then had his boots taken off and his feet soaked in hot water by the two or three 'servants' designated to serve him. I don't know if he was ever pulled up for it, or if this snob-quotient was considered essential, or adequate.

Our house in the plantations was the best we ever lived in, overlooking a sweeping green vista of cleanly cropped tea shrubs, with the mist-wrapped ranges of the Annamalais in the distance. I was entitled to a cook, a gardener, a sweeper, a butler, the butler's sidekick called 'boy' and a driver—all perquisites of my managerial status. Imagine Vijay and I living in this nannydom, constantly watched and fussed over, like kids in Victorian England. I brought the number down to three and was penalized, by being taxed for six. For a total of nine years, I paid tax for my liberty. Fair enough: I was breaking a norm to suit my needs, I was insisting on my freedom and why should that come free?

When Vijay's *Bihar Is in the Eye of the Beholder* was being edited, this guy, who worked for the publisher and is also a good friend, came over to stay. The editing went well. The evenings? With the writer and editor suitably lubricated, the food on the table hardly mattered which was great, for me. On the last night, our guest who could clearly see through my cooking dis-abilities declared that he would cook that night. He had a good hand for it too.

There was a club dinner to attend during his stay and we were to take him along. When I got back from work in the evening, Vijay pointed out a hitch: Our friend from Delhi happened to be wearing open shoes but the club required that you wear *proper* shoes—don't you know, with laces, and socks and all of that. Vijay's footwear size was 11 and our friend's a modest 7 or 8. We went, our guest wearing size 11 shoes with paper stuffed into the empty spaces. I remember the two of them positioned somewhere behind the bar-counter and behind their whisky-sodas. The Delhi feet were cleverly concealed.

My dislike for official dinners—which require equal proportions of sophistication and bluster—is a personality defect I am unable to rectify. The number of times I have given those dinners a miss is embarrassing. I had been hauled up for my absences, so I did make a genuine effort to go. My tested remedy for personal discomfiture is a glass of the needful. I counted on Vijay for this and he did not fail me even once, but soon after, he would do his magical vanishing act… I saw him now and then in the midst of dark-suited thicket of men around the bar which was okay as long as he stayed alert enough to drive us safely back home.

So my corporate years were an essential part of my education—socially, culturally and at work. The rigid hierarchy within the company was at times frustrating. There used to be an annual cultural event at which the managers competed with the staff in several sporting events. This was followed by high tea. Vijay who hated wearing a suit (he bought one second-hand, after I joined the company) was told by some managers that it was compulsory for the occasion. He wanted to know why, after all it was an informal event.

'It is the only day that we mingle with the staff socially,' a manager told him. 'To express our friendship. This dress code is just a subtle way of maintaining our distance.'

How much more subtle can you be?

The Tata Group is known to be one of the best, invariably several notches above most of their peers. Their welfare work in the plantations is praiseworthy. I was happy with being a surgeon handling the health care of a well-organized labour force and earned an Excellence Award from the company. But I was a misfit who lacked many of the social graces. I was the disjointed finger, the nail in the corporate shoe. Nevertheless, the nine years I spent working for the Tata Group* were a unique opportunity to manage the welfare of a large working community. I remain forever indebted.

*I worked for Tata Tea and then for Tata Coffee between 1998 and 2014, with a six-year intermission when we lived in Lonavla.

19

Home Building

Starting 2006, we lived in Lonavala in Maharashtra for six years. Its charm as a hideout and its nearness to Pune and Mumbai—each with its own piquant virtues—drew us away from the unruffled calm of the south. How bold, how foolish, how vitalizing a venture it would be, time would tell. Our two-bedroom corner-house on Sector E of Gold Valley was within touching distance of the mist-laden Sahyadris. In the next couple of years as more houses came up, we were in closer proximity to less attractive landscape. We witnessed the construction of houses up close. We ate, slept and dreamed to the music of drills, cement-mixers, water tankers and trucks plying building material. As dream homes such as ours came up, they wounded the landscape and mutilated nature. Within months, there was a shortage of water and unless you were prudent, buying it by the tanker was the only choice.

We were one of half a dozen full-time resident couples in the newly built housing society, living in quiet five days a week. The other house-owners were families from Pune and Mumbai who came on weekends, seduced by the exuberance of the hills and rains that were plentiful. The people of Lonavala tolerated them, wrested as much as they could out of their two-day splurge, and heaved a mighty sigh of relief when they left. They would come again, like a swarm of locusts, but in an entourage of vehicles. The water tankers plied endlessly, generators kicked in, hundreds of lights came on, speakers boomed music loud enough to keep the stars awake.

The construction workers lived in makeshift shacks right next to the houses that came up. The builders looked the other way as electric cables were tugged into place to provide single-bulb electricity to each shack. Water came from a borewell via hand pumps. The construction of two hundred and fifty Gold Valley homes was completed in April 2009 and the workers' homes were dismantled two days later. The supply of water and electricity were summarily cut off; the workers and their families were told to leave. Some went back to their villages; others set off in search of similar work. A small number found jobs in Gold Valley as security men, gardeners and domestic workers.*

A few months after we moved to Lonavla, I set up a clinic within the premises, about a kilometre from home. I got the room rent-free from the builders by reminding them that the health of the workers was a responsibility they had to fulfil, and that it could easily be done by giving me some space. Thereafter I frequented the office until they decided to take a chance and offered me a little room which I gladly accepted.

The patients were largely workers who migrated from the villages of Maharashtra and the districts of Bidar, Gadag, Gulbarga and Belgaum in Karnataka. I dispensed medicines and gave injections. The cost of treatment ranged from ten to thirty and occasionally fifty rupees. Sometimes one of the weekenders would turn up at the clinic and I would make a queenly sum.

I was in good cheer until I found that many of the workers

*There are several lakh construction workers who form the unorganized labour force in our country. They have no protection from the uncertainty of wages, poor living conditions or the sudden cessation of work. There is no welfare, there is no compensation.

preferred the doctors and quacks in town who offered instant cures. 'I want quick relief,' said one man who had come with a stomach ailment. 'I need injections. Or a drip.'* I explained that the real remedy was in improving the body's defences against disease. I spoke eloquently about hygiene and nutrition, and told him that I would hold meetings to explain healthy habits, distribute soaps and hand towels.

'It will be like shooting the tail of a rabid dog,' the man said, unenthused. 'We will fall ill over and over again. We always do. Just give me medicines so I can work.' I got his medicines ready. 'What to do, madam. We are dying...slowly dying...but we want to live.' He pocketed the medicines and left.

Ratna was a garrulous and cheery young woman who came twice a week to help in our home. She had studied for a year at the village school in Gadag before her father stopped her schooling so she could tend their goats. Eight years after her marriage to Mariappa (a seventh-class dropout), they came to Lonavala in search of work. Ratna was smarter than her husband and showed a great desire to learn. She asked innumerable questions and shared with me filmi gossip which she heard on television. Two years on, she could read and write fluently in Kannada and not-so fluently in Hindi and English. She credits me with the teaching, but most of her learning was on her own.

Ratna had questions. The lady who lived in her own bungalow down the road? She gave herself injections every morning after breakfast and then popped pills, Ratna said.

*One of the miracle injections so used is steroid combined with penicillin, a relief-package widely used by doctors and quacks. You can find them in every village, town and city of India. These practitioners continue to flourish right under the noses of our government officials. Along with a bottle of intravenous glucose it never fails to impress patients who have repeatedly told me that they feel their symptoms fade away and energy seep in. It is difficult to convince them about the dangers of such treatment. Steroids, arbitrarily used, weaken the bones, raise blood pressure and lower immunity. The overuse of antibiotics leads to the body becoming resistant to the drug if used for any future illness.

'Madam has the best home, best car, best food and everything. Then why does she fall ill?'

Not wanting to discuss the lady's problems, I said, 'You fall ill too. And you know why.'

She looked uncertain. 'You told me about germs that come from unclean hands and from water that is not boiled. But madam is very clean. She uses soap and Dettol and scented sprays.' Glumly she surveyed our home: 'Madam's is the best.'

She then made a telling observation about a health programme on television: 'They talk about exercises to do in front of the computer or sitting on a chair or when travelling in a car or aeroplane. I want to know what *I* must do to stop my back from hurting.'

'It's all the bending down to sweep and carrying buckets of water,' I said, wisely.

She frowned. 'That's what you ask me to do when I come here.'

Ratna's husband is a work-horse without much imagination, but wise enough to let his wife make the decisions that influence their future. They will one day live in a better home than the little shed they now live in. Her children will go to an English-medium school. If anyone can make it happen, it is Ratna.

*

So Vijay and I settled in and began to think of ourselves as locals. Friday was the big day of the week—for marketing. It was a ten-minute drive into town. The weekly purchase of victuals took up most of half a day. The kiraana first, with Vijay striking off items on the list while I pressed forward at the counter asking sharp questions; the Punjab Bakery next for bread, butter, jam, pickle and a few of my favourite buns; Madhukar Chemists; and then the vegetable market spread out over an open maidan on the edge of the town (the car slowing down on the way at the cinema house to check on the movie).

We carried four bags and made our way between vendors seated on the ground. After this, there would be the paying of telephone or electricity bills, the post office, the courier, a gas cylinder refill, haircuts and then the tea-break, with gulab jamun or samosas; sometimes a movie in the evening and then chicken curry for dinner and maybe sausages next morning. Very nice.

It was 2010. The monsoons were late by a month. Then the lashings began, and did not stop. As our house was on the lower end of a slope, we had water lapping at the gate. By the third day the gate was half under water. There was no real flaw in the system of storm-water drains which connected to a larger outlet, so the water streamed away in a gorge downhill. But the plastic and other garbage that were chucked indiscriminately by the residents had blocked the outlet. Basheer—the local handyman who looked after the plumbing, electricity and water supply—waded through knee-deep water to reach our gate. 'Water inside the electric box,' he said, indicating the lopsided contraption fixed a few feet away from our gate and now submerged. 'All your wiring comes through it…I'm not touching.' The worst-hit were the workers and their children because the danger from loose and dangling wires was very real. We pleaded with him to get some men who would help unblock the drains.

Late afternoon, two men came with shovels and set to work. Out came a heap of cola bottles, use-and-throw plates, cups, packets and empty plastic sacks used to carry cement. How many bags of cement go into constructing one house? Who is responsible in 'environment-friendly' housing societies (like ours) where the builders don't think it's their job to clear up after construction work?

The Residents' Association of Gold Valley had appealed to fellow residents about the dangers of throwing away garbage. Everyone assured us that they never 'chuck', but the majority did; or they left plastic bags filled with waste outside their gates where stray dogs tore them open and strewed the waste across the roads whereupon the strong hill winds carried them into the drains. This is a collective criminal activity enabled by the public and ignored by the concerned officials and medical professionals. Until matters come to a head, as it did in Pune.*

*See Chapter 25.

20

Rural Wounds, Urban Ulcers

In his essay 'How the Poor Die', George Orwell offers a look inside a common man's hospital in Paris. He was on a visit to the city in 1929 when he fell ill with pneumonia and was admitted to the hospital for several weeks. He describes the horrific indignities the poor were subjected to, and the tragedy of one who must die in such a hospital. The unclean toilets, the inefficient treatment and the indifference of doctors and nurses towards their patients shocked Orwell; at that time, England offered far better health care to the poor. But fifty years earlier, England too had been just as bad. In the 1850s, the English kept away from their shoddy hospitals, says Orwell, because they were more like the 'antechambers of the tomb'.

The scenes depicted in Orwell's essay are long past in France, but in India they are all too familiar. It hardly matters where you are in the country, just step out and exercise your eyes. One brief visit to the general ward of a government hospital will tell you everything. Many doctors work in their private clinics during official duty hours, while accepting a full salary with perks from the government. Some months ago, the owner of a coffee plantation had been nipped by a puppy. Since the pup died soon after, I advised him to take the anti-rabies vaccine, which had to be purchased, and costs over a thousand rupees. Government hospitals stock the vaccine for use on the general-ward category of patients. A week later when I met the planter, he said, 'I got the vaccine for free at the government hospital.' He went with a relative who spoke to the doctor who was a friend. He readily obliged, thus depriving some poor labourer with a dog bite who has neither a friend with influence nor the thousand bucks to pay for it.

That incident set me thinking: how do people from varied economic backgrounds manage when struck by a serious illness?

Kirpal Singh Mann ran Mann Auto Works near Aundh in Pune. He would be at work all day in his dusty garage from where he sells second-, third-and fourth-hand cars and two-wheelers after painting and patchwork. When we lived in Lonavla, we bought our WagonR from Kirpal Singh and since then he remained our car servicing agent-cum-advisor about all things Pune, like best-deal shops and restaurants. Since his wife was a Malayali, we could also ask him about the nearest paradise with porotta and chicken curry. The Manns were a modern, middle-class family with modern, middle-class ambitions. The wife dreamed of being able to go to her home in Kottayam every summer, bearing gifts for her people. Kirpal Singh was eyeing a Maruti 800 (in good health) that would make family outings more comfortable. Their only son who had landed his first job as a sales representative in a drug company was eager to save for a holiday in Singapore with friends.

Six months into his job, Kirpal's son got knocked down by a speeding truck while riding his motorbike on the Bombay-Pune Expressway. By the time his father got to the spot and rushed him to Bombay, six hours had elapsed. The young man had multiple fractures of his thigh bones and severe damage to the muscles and blood vessels. The orthopaedic department had no empty beds. Two pints of blood were transfused with the patient lying on a stretcher. By midnight he was given a bed in the general ward and operated soon after. Kirpal Singh ran around buying medicines. His son would need major surgery to fix the bones, two more pints of blood and hospital stay for two to three weeks. A deposit of Rs 30,000 and the second surgery next day. He left the hospital eighteen days later, on crutches. Total expenses: Rs 1,55,000. Since he was still on probation, his company would not reimburse his bills. But they let him have his job back when he went to work after six months. 'He's lucky to escape with his life,' the doctor replied when Kirpal Singh asked if there would be some concession on the bill.

In the year that followed there were hospital visits, medicines and physiotherapy, costing another Rs 50,000. All of this was somehow borne by this family of five (including Mann's parents) whose combined income was Rs 42,000 per month. They were not complaining. God had been good to them, he had saved their only son.

The Malwanis were a five-member family. The parents, son, his wife and the grandchild of seven years lived in Whispering Woods, a gated community in Ahmedabad. Father and son were in the footwear business and made a tidy sum between them. When the father had niggling chest pain and giddiness last year, they took him to the best private hospital where tests revealed a block in the blood supply to the heart. An angioplasty and unblocking of the artery was done next day for a cost of Rs 2,70,000. His comprehensive health insurance plan covered most of it; the illness did not make a dent on their savings. The Malwanis were satisfied and never failed to praise the doctors who made it possible for him to recover completely.

As daily wage-earners who built roads and worked at the brick kilns of Kurnool in Andhra Pradesh, Vishnu and Kalavathi were familiar with the harshness of penury. Kala had noticed a swelling on the side of her tongue for several months. She treated herself with more tobacco to alleviate the sharp twinges of pain besides soothing hunger which she dreaded more than the swelling on the tongue. Soon the pain became intolerable and she was spitting blood when Vishnu took her to the government hospital. After a week of being tossed around departments she landed at the cancer-detection clinic. Diagnosis: a malignant tumour exacerbated by the constant irritation of a carious tooth, and the effects of tobacco.

The doctors were angry with Kala for not reporting earlier. We could have cured you, they said. There was further delay while Vishnu paid a certain amount of money and purchased drugs. Days went by: a blood test one day, X-ray the next, and some days nothing but the wait. Three weeks after she had first entered the hospital, Kala started radiotherapy and injections. The swelling on her tongue shrank in size but in exchange she got nausea, vomiting and a raging fever. Vishnu brought milk, eggs and apples to revive her weakening body. Nothing worked. Kala, aged twenty-five, took her last breath less than two months after stepping into hospital. Her last wish? Please, some tobacco.

Vishnu did not escape the tragedy of Kala's illness: bouts of drinking and self-pity, suicidal urges and the neglect of their three children whose future had just got several shades darker followed.

Every one of us is a part of the system which makes it possible to have good medical care only if you have adequate financial resources. The fear of illness is universal and the Malwanis among us have the means for a quick and complete recovery, never mind the cost; the lower middle-class must face the added dangers of debt and the sudden emptying of life's savings; the daily wage-earner, the farm-hand, the destitute widow and the homeless are almost always defeated when struck by a serious illness. We are suitably proud of our clever doctors and the excellent hospitals which attract patients from other countries. We also need to be deeply ashamed of being able to help only a small fraction of our own people.

I have largely been unaware of the problems of urban welfare, particularly of the indigent people in our cities. Some years ago Vijay and I visited a slum in Chennai. As we stepped out of the autorickshaw a group of women approached us with affable curiosity. When we introduced ourselves (one doctor, one journalist) an alert, middle-aged maami said in a huff: 'We don't need more doctors.' She pointed across the road to a row of cubbyhole clinics with Red Cross symbols on their dust-laden doors. 'They bleed us, like mosquitoes.' At ten in the morning we were already being bled, by the insect variety. 'You people are in danger of falling ill with malaria,' I said, swiping daintily at a mosquito, then another and another. 'You *need* doctors.' She wasn't convinced. 'They treat us when we are ill, for what? Fall sick, take medicines, get better. Fall sick, take medicines, get better. We spend more money on tablets and injections than on food.'

A young man stepped into the conversation. 'This arm,' he said, displaying a twisted right elbow. 'Autorickshaw accident. The doctors at the hospital put a plate and many screws, and charged fifteen thousand. The wound started to pour pus. I swear I did not drink a drop of milk, or eat a single egg or banana, and still the pus. The doctors filled me up with their medicines. Every *oosi* cost hundred rupees or more. I had to sell my wife's earrings and two bangles. I went to another hospital and spent more…sold my rickshaw and pulled our three children out of school. Two months, sixty thousand rupees and a stiff arm. Light work is all I can do now.' He looked at his faded shorts and vest that looked like it had been ridden with bullets. 'I was a smart auto driver. Do you think the doctors used old screws taken out of someone who ended up in the grave?'

A discussion ensued. The three main scourges of the slum residents were malaria, diarrhoea and chest infections. The homes overlooked the banks of the Cooum River which flows through the city. The water was choked with the garbage and industrial debris. Further east, a sluggardly stream of filthy water mingled with the Cooum before it flowed into the sea. The stench was foul. Mosquitoes in thick clusters resided in their homes. Heavy traffic meant that the slum-dwellers breathed air poisoned with petrol and diesel fumes.

The doctors across the road were a busy lot. If patients asked questions, they were admonished severely: 'Drink only boiled water,' 'Don't smoke,' 'Keep your children clean,' the doctor said, scribbling her multi-drug prescription. A visit to one of these private clinics cost two to three hundred rupees, sometimes more. A day's wages.

Invariably, inside every tarpaulin-corrugated-metal-and-plastic home that was roughly five to six paces square, was a fan resting on bare ground, a naked bulb overhead and several dangling wires. (Electricity was illegally procured.)

'We don't mind the stench,' a woman explained, scratching herself as she spoke, 'if we could be rid of the mosquitoes. A fan helps more than anything else.' 'Anything else' were agarbattis that were mostly useless, or tubes of insect repellent which cost forty-five rupees and lasted only a few days for a family.

Outside this huddle of homes a group of women sat in a circle, sorting out what looked like the bones of some animal. A closer look and we knew it to be a large animal, a buffalo or a cow. 'We get them from the slaughter house,' explained one of the women. 'Cheap and very good when added to any gravy, especially when there is some boti (entrails) to throw in.' Did they also eat the meat? 'Meat? Of course. At marriage feasts.'

It was a small slum of a hundred homes and eight hundred to a thousand people. At ten in the morning the only residents we could meet were those who did not go out to work: the pre-school children, the old and the disabled. Even among these, I picked up a number of skin infections, signs of anaemia and malnutrition. I considered visiting my medical brethren across the road. But anything that I said would be interference. Good sense prevailed and we went back to the hotel. I remember saying to some of the folk who saw us off. 'Don't worry. We will do something about this.'

It was an empty promise. I did nothing.

The way we live cheek to cheek with filth is the worst horror I know. The fact that some of us are able to seek out good health facilities with our wealth while leaving the poor to suffer inexorable hardships is the worst terror I know. An unspoken crime, the brutality of which lies in its indifference.*

The Chennai slum taught me more than a year's worth of lectures on community health at medical college. There are slums as big as Dharavi in Mumbai, and those as small as the one we went to in Chennai. Thirty to forty per cent of the people with whom we share our cities have no choice but to live in plastic shacks that they tack to whatever wall or tree will offer support; or on the pavement. Where is the water supply, where are the toilets, drainage and electricity? How do they manage the rains, the flooding and the occasional cyclones? Rooftops are blown away, homes crumple and die while their inhabitants run for their lives. Slums are the concentration camps of our country where disease and pollution do the killing.† That night in Chennai, I dreamt of a slum walking behind me on so many legs, hundreds of dwellings lurching, swaying and shuddering in pursuit as I fled.

*

*It would be unfair to bypass the small percentage of society which fights against the perplexing laws of iniquity; individuals, organizations, hospitals and even pockets within the benumbed governmental systems which work towards erasing these monstrous flaws. One example that comes to mind is Wenlock Hospital in Mangalore, Karnataka.

†The prime minister has declared that he will ensure the eradication of tuberculosis in India by 2025. In 2018, 4.2 lakh Indians coughed their way to the cemetery or the crematoria. If our PM fulfils his promise, he will be the sorcerer to beat all those who came before him.

I have been to New York twice, with the grand interval of thirty years between them. An evening on my first visit we drove through a locality where vacant-eyed men, mainly Blacks, were seated along the kerb, watching the cars drive past. Behind them were 'twenty-four-hour' booze shops lit up with neon lights. In the shadows, squalor.

'This is Harlem,' said my friend who was at the wheel. We were on our way to dinner at the house of a neurosurgeon, and we mentioned Harlem. Our host was somewhat dismissive. 'It's a wretched *slum*, that's what it is. The depressed classes—mainly immigrants and Blacks—live in Harlem.'

Slums in New York? I was curious.

'It's pure laziness. Give a Black man the bottle, and he's happy until it's empty. Then he will beg or steal to get another. If it's not drink, it's drugs.'

'I wish they would go back to their own countries,' said his wife.

Her husband gave an elaborate account of their egregious habits and their utter disregard for discipline. 'There have been efforts to integrate the Blacks and other immigrants with the rest of us. It won't work. They are a different species. We have to keep our distance. Especially for the sake of our children.'

We sat down to a wonderful dinner of spring chicken, individually cooked, and served with an exotic vegetable, either asparagus or artichoke. I was struggling with what I had just heard. 'Whatever the differences, they should not be living like that.' I persisted.

The doctor put down his knife and fork; he cleared his throat of annoyance. 'Have you heard of bussing? No? Bussing is a new strategy that is being introduced in the education system. To *ensure* segregation of people, you know—the different sections of society. School buses will take Black children to specified zones where there are schools for them. They will get a good education, and our children will not have to mix with them.'

His tall, serious, spectacled figure and his name spring to mind. He was a Cuban, for heaven's sake, his parents emigrated when he was fifteen.

'Let them be comfortable in their neighbourhoods and we will be happy in ours,' said his wife. 'More chicken?'

Thirty years later I was in New York, for a book-reading at Columbia University. I was rather excited and it went well, but at the back of my mind was a practical problem: the suitcase which had seen me through my trip was broken. I asked about a nearby shop where I could buy a new bag but an inexpensive one. My host caught on.

'I'll send a nice young Spanish guy from our office to go with you,' she said. 'He'll know best.' The first thing I said to the Spanish guy was, 'Will you take me to Harlem?'

A dark brown eyebrow did a leap and plunge. 'Sure?'

'Yes. I heard it's just walking distance from here. It's sure to have bargain shops.'

'Nothing but,' he grinned. 'Come along.'

Why Harlem, he asked me as we walked down an incline. I told him about my first visit, and about wanting to see what changes might have taken place since.

He was silent for a while before he spoke. 'I came to this country seven years ago. Lived on one of these streets for eighteen months with friends who arrived a year earlier.'

We kept walking. Just few minutes away was the university where some of the best minds in the world come together, a hallowed grove of many a Nobel winner. I was used to rubbing elbows with squalor in India but to see it in the US was like finding a cockroach in the soup at a Buckingham Palace dinner. ('We are not pleased.')

Broken pavements, overflowing waste bins, and the passers-by, mostly people of colour, emaciated or grossly over-weight. We entered a shop that sold everything. I found a suitcase for ten dollars but when it came to the payment counter, I noticed that it had been changed for a smaller one. The guy tried to get away by insisting that it was the one I chose. I stuck my ground, the manager came along and the bigger suitcase was quickly handed over. Walking back, I asked my escort what he felt about Harlem.

'You have to get out of here quick or you're cooked. Poverty grabs you by the balls...Hey, you and I are outsiders, you know. We don't ask questions.'

A couple of days later on the flight back home, I was talking to a fellow Indian who worked in New York. I told him about my visit to Harlem.

'It's like this,' he explained, with great seriousness. 'When there is menial work of any sort to be done, it is the lowest common denominator that does it.'

'Which—lowest common denominator?'

'The Blacks. TheMulattos. TheHispanics. Poor Bangladeshis and maybe some Indians. Slums are a part of development. I live in an upmarket area. But on my way to work, I have to go past Harlem. The no-good bums who resort to crime and lawlessness live in there. When down and out, they take up any sort of work, for any salary. When a small cafe needs a cook or waitress, a shop or office needs a cleaner or the drains need unblocking, they're ready. These jobs are always temporary, so when they lose their jobs they stick around with the hope of finding another. They gravitate to where others like them live and that's how slums are created. Crime is never far from the minds of slum-dwellers. Given the chance...'

What was to be done?

'Create new districts adjoining each city where they can live, give them transport to come to work, and then let them cope,' he said, with conviction.

I should forgive him his short-sighted comments. He is one of those unfortunate bankers who understands money, not life.

21

Doctoring Reality

Keeping a promise I made to myself years ago, I write this chapter about a few of my heroes in the medical field.

In the 1960s, Jagdish and Shipra Banerjee went to the UK for postgraduate studies in surgery and anaesthesia. When they came back, they were expected to rise quickly in their chosen fields. It was the 1970s and Delhi was a city of promise for top-quality professionals. Declining offers from the best hospitals, the Banerjees set up Rural Medicare Centre in the outskirts of Delhi, surprising everyone and disappointing many. Having keenly observed the needs of those who lived in a dusty backyard of the national capital, they figured out their act.

I first met the Banerjees at a conference of rural surgeons in Vapi, Gujarat, in 2002. A few years later I visited their hospital, the Rural Medicare Centre, modest and unremarkable in appearance with cramped wards separated into curtained cubicles. Each cubicle had just enough space for a bed, a locker, intravenous drip-stand and a stool for the attender. Amidst the clatter and chaos of hospital activity, the nurses and doctors moved between patients, working amidst the frenetic commotion of difficult medical situations. The hospital is known for top-quality treatment and is affordable for the average Indian: a rare virtue, you will notice, no matter where you go in our country. To work at Rural Medicare is a matter of pride. Three of the doctors I met—a surgeon, an obstetrician and an ophthalmologist—have stayed on for decades, in spite of more lucrative jobs available to them in the heart of Delhi.

I asked Shipra how a hospital such as theirs managed to tackle serious cases and perform major surgeries while financially keeping their heads above water. We were standing in a small reception area which buzzed with activity. It was early July and Delhi was on the boil.

'We stick to the essentials, and never let expenditure exceed income.'

'It cannot be easy to work in such conditions,' I said. 'It's so very hot…'

'We have fans!' Shipra exclaimed, pointing to a pensionable relic spinning overhead. She was a small sharp woman with a girlishness which belied her grit. 'I object to air conditioners, except in the operating theatre. Our patients are not used to them. And you know, our prices are fabulously low!' Then she added, with great seriousness: 'It is the lower middle-class and the impoverished who come to us. Our job is to be worthy of them.'

That's ambition.

Most hospitals in the country are unable to retain talented doctors on a fixed salary How were they able to manage? 'We work as equals,' said Shipra. 'Each one brings his or her skills and ideas. We provide the essentials and then work together. That's all we do.'

Dr Banerjee is a founder-member of the Association of Rural Surgeons of India (ARSI). It comprises a spirited group of surgeons who have built their careers in some of the remote, backward parts of the country. The original gang of about eight or twelve men and women who came together were from Midnapore in Bengal, Dondaicha in Maharashtra, Shimoga in Karnataka, Sivakasi in Tamil Nadu, and joined later by others from Orissa, Jammu and Kashmir, Himachal Pradesh, Gujarat,

Bihar and other states. Many have aged; a few have passed on. These doctors are a spirited lot and progressive in the best way possible. ARSI now has about thousand members. The annual conference, held in a different part of India every year, is a platform for the exchange of experience and innovation. The concept of using mosquito-netting as mesh for hernia repair (instead of the much more expensive marketed variety) is one such modernism being used widely, with complete safety. Problems of great magnitude faced by rural surgeons are addressed at the conference, such as the need to permit fresh blood transfusions in rural areas and the need to train young surgeons with broad-based surgical capabilities. The decision not to take the sponsorship of drug companies means that ARSI members fund their own travel and accommodation to attend the conference. Many of our neighbouring countries and others from Africa and Europe evinced interest in ARSI and so it went international. Dr Banerjee served as the President of ARSI for several years while Shipra, as a member of the governing council, has been actively involved all along. They retired from the Rural Medicare Centre some years ago, leaving an invaluable legacy in hospital care that none of the twinkling speciality hospitals which surround it can match.

*

Regi and Lalitha George are an unlikely couple: he is a Syrian Christian and she a seasoned bharatanatyam dancer and conservative brahmin who turns pale at the mention of meat curry. They met during their medical college years in Kottayam, Kerala, where Regi was general secretary and Lalitha the secretary of the Students' Union. Regi says it was her dazzling smile which first attracted him. When they got talking, he found they shared the same concerns about the medical system, and a daredevil spirit of adventure. They married soon after taking their degrees and for some years worked at a hospital in Tamil Nadu while dreaming of setting up their own. They travelled, in order to find a suitable place. The quiet hill-country of Sittilingi, a small rural town in Dharmapuri district of Tamil Nadu, seemed ideal. The land was lush, but without modern farming techniques or education, the farmers and the tribals of the area lived in penury and neglect. Medical facilities were non-existent.

Regi and Lalitha bought some land, built a thatch-roofed, one-room dispensary and opened the door to patients. At first the women came, with pregnancy and childbirth problems; then the children with stomach and chest ailments; and lastly the men, who were at first suspicious of the young couple. Within years the dispensary grew into a hospital with twenty beds, a laboratory, X-ray and a single-room operating theatre. Lalitha trained a dozen local girls in nursing and operating-room techniques, the sterilization of instruments, the taking of X-rays and doing simple blood tests. As natives of the area, these girls could relate well to the local population.

Regi, besides his medical and surgical work, took charge of administration and recruited a few young men. The office, housed in a couple of rooms set a few feet away from the wards, is a marvel. There is one desktop computer perched on a table, and a chair on which a staffer may sit to type or to take prints. At all other times, every one of the office staff and Regi sit cross-legged on the floor and work on their ledgers or laptops. It is the usual 8 a.m. to 5 p.m. office work. Regi says that the funds required to run such an institution will come, if the records are accurately maintained and the work audited. In the early years of their endeavour, he used to do all the leg-work that was required to make it happen. I did a six-week stint at the hospital when Regi and Lalitha took a much-needed holiday, and I used to try working in the office. Sitting cross-legged, I could barely manage two to three hours.

At the outpatient clinic in Sittilingi, there are 100 to 140 patients to be seen every day. In addition, there are surgeries, serious emergencies, accidents and night-calls. Sittilingi does not have a hospital within practical travelling distance for a sick villager. Salem is four hours by road and Bangalore five. The villagers are a hardy lot but their health has been damaged by the careless hand of globalization. Whatever was envisioned when that word was coined, it has come to mean a fog of uniformity propagated by corporate cunning, technology and advertisements. It brought processed food into humble homes while snatching away the nutritionally adequate diet of grains and pulses. Regi speaks of how the tribals of Sittilingi were coerced to give up their millet-rich diet: 'The ads that sell coloured soft drinks, noodles, biscuits and sweets are now screaming on television, which, ironically, are given as free gifts by the government. Empty starch, unhealthy fats, sugar and colouring agents have replaced the grains and pulses which the locals grew. It is hardly surprising that women in their seventies have naturally black hair and strong white teeth while their children and grandchildren are sickly and balding with weak bones and dental caries.'

With the advent of television, suicide rates among the youth increased. During my brief spell at Sittilingi I saw two or three every week, usually having taken the deadly pesticide compound of organo-phosphorus, used freely all over India to protect crops from insects. It is possible to save such patients if they are brought early. A stomach-wash to pump out the poison followed by atropine injections which serve as antidote will cancel the toxic effects. Many, however, reach too late. Among the other more deadly poisons are herbicide used to kill weeds, and kerosene. Neither has an antidote, and their consumption is often fatal.

Why the suicides? It is a pattern seen in our hinterlands and rarely highlighted by the medical world. My own observation while treating survivors of suicide attempts in Bihar, Uttar

Pradesh, Tamil Nadu and in my own Kodagu district of Karnataka revealed this: the young are being fed images of sleek urban youth with impossibly glamorous lifestyles. They try to imitate them, spending money they do not have to try and improve their appearances. Priorities get mixed up. They feel helpless, unable to break out of their worlds and into the glossy other-world of cars, fashion, glamour and glitz they see on screen. This gives way to depression, anger and resentment. Some turn criminals and indulge in burglary, rape and murder. Some turn the anger on themselves and try to commit suicide. Their actions are the outcome of a grossly unequal society: the emergency call for help.

A farmer's cooperative initiated by Regi has over a hundred farmers using organic methods to grow millets of many varieties, mustard, turmeric, groundnut and rice. Lalitha started a handicrafts unit and trained local women in tailoring and creating handmade articles that are suitable for sale. Along with organic produce from the co-operative farms, these are marketed and sold in the cities, fetching handsome profits for the villagers.

The hospital has a community-style kitchen for the staff. The doctors eat a meal or two every day in the common dining area next to the kitchen, mingling with the nurses and everyone else. Floor seating and steel plates for all, and a lot of chatter. I well recall the excellent food and the easy hospitality. ('Doctor, you like the kolambu? Take more, take more!')

Regi and Lalitha put their two sons through non-formal schooling for several years after which they went to J Krishnamurty's Rishi Valley School, in Madanapalli, Andhra Pradesh. Their schooling in the early years, from home, received help from Anuradha and Krishna, another couple who discovered Sittilingi around the same time as the doctors. Krishna is an engineer and Anuradha is an architect. Their objective was to help educate children who did not go to school. They taught their own two boys, and the doctors' kids joined them. All four have turned out to be excellent in their chosen fields: mathematics, medicine, liberal arts and history.

Anuradha helped design the house for Regi and Lalitha. Made of the rust-coloured laterite stones, the house encloses a garden and pond. Stone platforms substitute as beds, shelves and tables. It is a house so hospitable that scorpions, snakes and other like-minded creatures pay regular visits. Vijay and I lived there for those six weeks when I worked and one day witnessed the eye-popping spectacle of a battle between a well-muscled cobra and Caesar, the in-house Alsatian. The cobra turned tail and climbed up a mango tree, Caesar hurled canine abuses from below while Vijay implored him to leave the terrified adversary well alone. Cleopatra (Caesar's mate; of course) and I were reduced to being spectators. The drama that ensued ended with the terrified snake attempting an escape by coming down from the tree and next thing, Caesar was running amok with the snake twitching between his jaws. Vijay did his samurai thing with a stick and finally managed to relieve the sorry-looking mortal coils of the poor snake. Caesar wasn't too great for the rest of the day and we were worried until he licked up some breakfast next morning. We had another dramatic encounter with a scorpion in the kitchen but we will let that be.

The Sittilingi experiment continues to evolve. The hospital organizes an annual retreat for all their staff—a three-day event when they sit together and reflect on their work and objectives. They also have their work appraised by the patients and the local community. The rural surgeons' conference last year was held in Dimapur, Nagaland. Both Regi and Lalitha were busy and sent their young surgical colleague along. From what is said about his work and from the way in which he spoke about Sittilingi, it is clear that he has strengthened Regi and Lalitha's enterprise. What's more, a handful of young doctors have been motivated to work in rural hospitals in other states.

*

It was the swinging sixties when for the young, style meant at least as much as intellect. We were school-fresh, shy, insecure medics, all. One among us—gangling, spectacled sixteen-year-old Ravi Narayan from an Iyer family—stood out because of his maturity and composure that was way ahead of his sixteen years. His natural inclination was to eschew fashion; he was never with the rest of us who lined up outside movie theatres to watch the hottest and best. Ravi was no spoilsport, he was certainly not averse to mischief, within limits. We counted on him as a friend who would mediate with the authorities in times of trouble. His neatly written lecture notes were frequently borrowed; his opinion sought on almost everything.

In our batch of fifty medics, everyone was an achiever. But some achieved more than the others. Ravi stayed among the top few in the batch right through the academic years. After college, as I ploughed through my own choppy life, we remained friends. He is now grey-haired and a little less slim, but youthful and fervent in the pursuit of his goals. A few months ago, having warned Ravi and his wife Thelma that I would be devouring several hours of their time, I landed up at their home in Koramangala, Bangalore.

It is believed that 70 per cent of what we become is because of inherited genetic factors. Environment shapes the remaining 30 per cent. In the early 1940s, Ravi's father was one of the first chartered accountants to establish practice in Lahore. He moved to Delhi with his newly wedded wife just before Partition and died of a heart attack when Ravi was nine. The young widow found work with Kamaladevi Chattopadyay, the pioneer of India's handicrafts industry and a veritable leader in the forefront of national politics. Impressed by the young Mrs Iyer's clear-sightedness and sharp intellect, Kamaladevi asked her if she would like to take active part in politics. She declined and chose instead to head the handicrafts sector in Bangalore. The family moved from Delhi and Ravi joined St John's Medical College soon after school.

I said to Ravi that even as a teenager, I had been curious about his capacity for restraint and perseverance. 'My mother was a resourceful woman,' he reflected. 'She found it hard to manage her work and bring up her children. Instead of hiring an assistant to help with her job, she asked my elder brother and me, and later my sister, to help. We typed letters, received phone calls, managed incoming and outgoing mail and kept accounts. We learnt the meaning of responsibility at a young age.'

During his internship, Ravi found that he disliked hospital practice: the severe, almost punitive manner of medical therapy, the over-reliance on diagnostic aids, the theoretical hyperbole about technical progress and the shift towards remote-control medicine never attracted him. The college dean, worried that one of his brightest pupils was losing his mind, sent him to the psychiatrist.

It was 1971, the year of the crisis in East Pakistan and the creation of Bangladesh. Faced with a serious shortage of medical personnel and medicines, the country accepted aid and volunteers from India. Ravi was one among eight interns (including two nuns) from our batch who opted to work in Bangladesh during their internship. It was rich experience.

Rural posting, meant to help us understand the importance of community health, had pushed me in the opposite direction, for I found it dull and uninspiring. Much later I was to hear from Ravi how the unique experience in trying to impart medical wisdom to people ravaged by war had helped him find his own direction. In the early days of the posting in Bangladesh, Ravi was told to take charge of an impending delivery. The patient stood leaning against the wall of her hut. 'Easy case,' the doctor had snapped when the intern tried to articulate his inexperience. 'This is her fourth delivery.' Nervously trying to recollect the process of bringing a baby into the world, Ravi directed her to lie down on the cot. 'Whoever heard of such a thing?' she exclaimed, and lowered herself to a squatting position. 'The baby will find it easier this way.' She delivered safely, within the hour. 'There are many seriously ill patients who need your help,' she said, smiling at the astonished intern. 'I can manage.' Years later we find that many obstetricians have switched to delivering babies in the squatting position, with gravity assisting the mother and the baby.

The biggest lesson he learnt during his rural posting was that patients are often wiser than doctors assume. They need to be listened to. When he returned, Ravi was as confused as ever but had one resolve. He would opt out of hospital practice and pursue his interest in tropical medicine and community health, both of which had few takers among young doctors. Who wants to spend a lifetime studying lesser known evils like kaalaazaar, leptospirosis or eichinococcus? Who wants to write academic papers about sewage plants and septic tanks? Ravi did.

He studied tropical medicine in London, came back to the college and worked in community health. He started to motivate and guide many of the younger doctors. Among them was Thelma Rodrigues.

To many of the village folk who came to hospital, Thelma was the 'bob-cut doctor'. During her internship and the rural posting to some villages near Bangalore she thought nothing of hitching rides on lorries, trucks and bikes in order to reach the dusty outskirts of the city. The villagers were bewildered by her boldness; Ravi, the staid Iyer boy, was intrigued. A unique sort of girl, this: she challenged his chivalrous nature by refusing to have doors opened or books carried for her.

Thelma belongs to a family of historic import. Her grandfather operated one of the earliest postal services in villages adjoining Bhopal, carrying post in mule carts! It served well for a long time, right until the Post and Telegraph department reached the hinterlands. His son, Joe Rodrigues, was a naval recruit who, inspired by Subash Chandra Bose, later joined the Indian National Army (INA). He became one of the five trusted aides of Bose, in charge of ambush attacks on British forces. When Bose died and the INA was dismantled, Joe Rodrigues was arrested along with the others who had been in the forefront of INA. A high-profile trial followed. If it wasn't for a bright young lawyer named Jawaharlal Nehru who fought their case, they would have been hanged. Joe Rodrigues subsequently joined the Indian Police Service and had a distinguished career.

How could the daughter not turn out to be bold as well as courageous? The 'bob-cut doctor' married the Iyer* after an initial period of resistance from the Catholic church. Ravi, in his usual style, persisted in talking to the Jesuit priests and the bishop until he convinced them. Ravi and Thelma founded SOCHARA—a highly acclaimed institution for training in community-based health and research. It has subsidiary centres in Bangalore, Bhopal and Chennai. Through its many activities, SOCHARA has succeeded in highlighting defects in our health system, stressing the importance of medical ethics and influencing major health policies in the country while helping doctors to choose their career paths wisely. The contribution of this couple towards public health is immeasurable.

*

Speaking of my idols, I can hardly leave out the two remarkable 19th-century champions of hand washing.

In my early years of training, the washing of hands before an operation ranged from a carefree slapping of a cake of soap between the hands and spraying some water, to a compulsive fifteen-minute scrub up to the elbows or the armpit. Some surgeons believed in a more meticulous preparation,

*Ravi's grandfather had decided to do away with 'Iyer' as his surname because of its caste significance

by taking a preoperative shower or bath. Older hospitals in many countries provide bathing facilities within the operating-theatre complex. An American surgeon told me he jogs five kilometres to the hospital, takes a shower and then sets upon his patients.

In Liverpool hospitals, the scrubbing took a good ten minutes. The professor, assistants and scrub nurse lined up before a long trough with taps fitted on the wall along its front. Containers with antiseptic scrubbing lotion attached near each tap dripped the stuff into your hands as you soaped to the elbows and scrubbed with a brush, the ten-minute drill leavened by chit-chat. The players were English, Irish, Welsh, Scottish, Nigerian, Maltese, Egyptian, Ugandan, Sri Lankan, Burmese, Australian and Indian. A colourful team we were, pink, brown, black and yellow, scrubbing away layers of healthy epidermis, fighting off the germs. (Subsequently I have found that a two-minute cleanse with our own cheapest-and-best, friendly pink Lifebouy works just as well.) With all the punishment from years of scrubbing, my hands turned rough while those of my pen-holding husband stayed soft. That's so unfair.

The history of hand washing, so essential to the healer and the healed, begins with Ignaz Semmelweis, a Hungarian born in 1818. He took his medical degree from Vienna and joined the General Hospital as an assistant surgeon in Obstetrics. He was to teach medical students, supervise deliveries and keep clinical records in the maternity department. Infanticide was not uncommon among unwed mothers and prostitutes. The hospital therefore offered free childbirth service and childcare benefits to needy mothers. Patients admitted in Clinic 1 were managed by trainee doctors and medical students; in Clinic 2 they were under the care of midwives.

The death rate among women who delivered in Clinic 1 (10 to 30 per cent) was much higher than in Clinic 2 (4 per cent). The maternity wards became places to dread and women preferred to deliver at home or even on the streets. Those who came to hospital pleaded, on bended knees, for Clinic 2. According to the medical wisdom of the times, 'child-bed fever' which caused death after delivery was due to unclean bowels. Women were given purgatives before delivery to cleanse their system. Poorly functioning kidneys, wrong diet, emotional disturbance and pressure on the womb from the growing foetus were also held responsible. Some blamed an imbalance of humours and still others claimed that unfavourable atmospheric-cosmic-terrestrial influences (termed miasma) led to the deaths. The mystery remained.

Semmelweis was confounded by the differential mortality between the two clinics of the same hospital. On checking procedural details, he found that doctors went back and forth between the autopsy rooms and the maternity wards—*from the dead to the living*—as a part of their training. One day a doctor accidentally cut his finger while doing an autopsy and it became septic. Could it be some cadaveric particles that caused the sepsis? What if the maternity deaths in Clinic 1 were the result of a cadaveric poison transmitted by the medics? In Clinic 2 the midwives who conducted the deliveries had nothing to do with the dead.

Semmelweis instructed his students to wash their hands in chlorinated lime before attending childbirth. This was strictly followed by his juniors for two months, from April to June of 1847. The mortality rate in Clinic 1 dropped from 18 per cent to 2 per cent within two months and in less than a year it was negligible. The young doctor had uncovered an elementary truth: cleanliness reduces infections.

The triumphant young doctor conveyed his finding to his seniors, the professors of obstetrics. Every one of them ridiculed, rejected or ignored it. Semmelweis wrote letters and articles explaining the need for hand hygiene and the cleaning of instruments used in delivery. Within a year, his job was terminated as punishment for defiant behaviour. He found a job in Budapest but no support for his cause. He took to writing bitter, angry letters to obstetricians all over Europe, exhorting them to accept the truth of his findings. Medical men and scientists of the highest authority (James Young Simpson and Virchow among them) were not convinced. Semmelweis became depressed, his personal life suffered. He might have developed early dementia or late-stage of syphilis but that is mere conjecture. (It was still not known that syphilitic mothers whose deliveries the doctors conducted, could infect them and Semmelweis could have been one such victim.) His mood swings and irrational behaviour could just as easily have been due to the ridicule and unfair persecution by the medical fraternity. He was duped into visiting a mental asylum and once inside, put in solitary confinement. Brutally beaten up by the guards, he died fourteen days after entering the asylum when infection of his wounds led to septicaemia.

Within a decade, the work of Louis Pasteur and Joseph Lister proved the truth of his findings. Minute germs that cause disease were found in the environment and on human skin. The need to wash one's hands to prevent infection is now the chartbuster among the many commandments of preventive health care.

It is difficult to imagine that the concept of cleanliness is so recent, as we learn from Orwell's account of a hospital in Paris in 1929. People in colder countries bathed only when body odour forced them to face the exertion, no more than a few times a year. In England people waited for the warm month of May to peel off their clothes and subject the body to a full bath. Weddings were held in the summer months and the custom of the bridal bouquet ensured a sweet-smelling bride. Henry Thoreau, who did a brief stint as a schoolteacher in Concord in the US in 1837, left in disgust because of two things he abhorred: the tradition of corporal punishment, and the windowless classrooms which smelled foul by the end of the day.

*

Born to a wealthy English family in 1820 (two years after Semmelweis), Florence Nightingale was as bright as she was determined. She made good use of the classical education she received at a time when girls merely looked forward to making a good marriage. Florence did not want a domesticated life and turned down a suitor, in spite of his being to her romantic and intellectual liking. To her disappointed father she explained that she would rather put her life to some good use instead of 'whiling it away serving sumptuous teas to wealthy have-alls in a dainty parlour'. Instead, she opted to spend two years in Germany to learn nursing.

Florence returned to England after the training and joined a hospital on Harley Street. She also volunteered at Middlesex Hospital where her work in improving hygiene during a cholera outbreak reduced the number of deaths to a large extent. In 1853 the war in Crimea broke out; within a year, 18,000 soldiers were admitted to the hospital where facilities were poor. The government had to take quick action. In 1854, Sidney Herbert who was the secretary of war wrote to Florence Nightingale asking if she could take a team of nurses to the base hospital in Constantinople. She would be given full control of the operations. Within weeks, Florence gathered three dozen volunteers and set sail to the Black Sea.

In Crimea she truly understood the appalling consequences of war and the fate of its casualties. The base hospital in Scutari was built on a swamp, with dirty water seeping into the building. The medical personnel were few and overworked, the hospital was filthy; patients with festering wounds and gangrenous limbs lay upon beds soiled with their own excreta. Water was so scarce, even drinking water had to be rationed.

Rodents, ticks and fleas kept the soldiers company. Every day, the dead were carried away in cartloads to the morgue.

'Brushes!' she said. 'Hundreds of brushes. And soap!' The wards were scrubbed from floor to roof, the linen was washed in boiling water, the cots scraped of dirt and the windows opened wide to let the sunlight in. Patients were bathed, fed, and their wounds dressed, with soldiers who were not too infirm helping the nurses. Outcome: the luxury and the dignity of cleanliness; less suffering and better rates of cure. In the eighteen months that she spent in Crimea, Florence Nightingale transformed the very nature of health care and reduced the mortality rate of the soldiers by 60 per cent.

She returned home to a hero's welcome. Queen Victoria gifted her a jewelled brooch and 250,000 pounds. She used the money to set up St Thomas Hospital, and a school of nursing. The US government asked her advice in improving the military hospitals during the Civil War. Although she never visited India, she did give proposals regarding community health in our country.

While in Crimea, at a young age, she contracted brucellosis, a lingering bacterial infection, and never fully recovered from it. She lived to be ninety but was house-bound and bedridden for most of her last fifty years and yet made good use of her experience to write books on nursing care. When Florence Nightingale died, the family abided by her wish that her funeral be modest and turned down the honour of a national funeral. The Lady with the Lamp was buried at a quiet ceremony in her family cemetery.

Such a life. Thanks to this remarkable woman, nursing became the foundation for patient care in hospitals. Doctors had gained their most trustworthy (and underrated) of colleagues. The contributions of Florence Nightingale to the medical world are as significant as any great scientific discovery or invention.

*

It is difficult to draw a straight line with life's purpose. Mine has been slanting, wobbly, even jagged in places. I get where I want to be, but the pot of water I carry spills a fair bit on the way. These heroes of mine have walked the straight line and delivered their pots of water. Maybe a few drops were spilt but most of it reached. These are tough acts to follow. And yet we have hundreds like them who have shown that the thoroughly messed-up wires of our medical system need to be simply and methodically laid out in order to work.

22
My Clinic

At a certain stage in my life, half-heartedly contemplating retirement, I realized that a life of surgery in far-flung places had enriched my mental arsenal adequately. It was time to assess my faculties in a new way. So after a long career of wielding the sharps, I disarmed myself. The time was ripe for a different kind of risk.

Had I the grit to survive without a support-team? I set up trade as a general practitioner in my home district of Kodagu in a rented room in Ponnampet, a two-street town 5 kilometres from our home. It is a curious little sub-municipality, with a statue of my grandfather's great-grandfather standing in the heart of the town. Cheppudira Dewan Ponnappa was one of the two trusted ministers to the erstwhile king who was deposed by the British in 1834.*

I furnished the room with a table, chairs, shelves, an examination couch and a calendar on a nail. That my clinic was between two barber shops was a fitting reminder of my surgical ancestry—the first association of surgeons of England having evolved from the barbers' guild. My clipper-sporting

*It is always better to take everything you hear or read about the antecedents of my people with an ample measure of salt. We are as good at fooling people as we are at being fooled. Our legendary and robust longevity is said to be due to such inherited gifts.

co-workers come to me with their medical problems, refer their clients and at times keep guard when I need to use the only toilet in the building complex (the door-latch doesn't work). In exchange I inveigled my husband into having his hair shorn by one and then the other. This professional friendship with barbers pleases me no end. I am as anxious for their trade to thrive as I am for mine. We have not borrowed tools from each other, though. Not yet.

The medicines I use are few and inexpensive. I make up for this thrift with advice: about food habits, exercise, hygiene and the reduction of stress-levels. I am listened to politely; or with dismay; or amusement. A few follow my counsel. My regulars tend to leave their personal belongings in the waiting area which is a cubicle with chairs and a side-table stacked with old magazines. They finish their purchase of provisions, visit the bank, the post office, bakery or one of the four liquor shops before returning to collect their articles. The other day a woman paused to show me a 'blouse-piece' she had purchased. Would it match her mango-green sari? On a busy day, the waiting-room resembles a bus stop with umbrellas, carry-bags, paper packets, helmets and on rare occasions a child or two, quietly tearing bits of paper or indulging in other wickedness until a parent or grandparent comes to claim them.

I am a grumpy user of the telephone. Happy were the days in Bihar and in Vrindavan where the intercom served to connect us with the hospital. We booked trunk-calls on urgent occasions and really, how much of living is urgent? With the entry of the cell phone (for us in 2009), life got more difficult. There is a sudden need to wish people on birthdays and anniversaries. And it takes some hard work to not know who met who the previous week. The phone itself is 'mobile' but it congeals the user in more ways than one. We doctors have it doubly hard, you see. 'Are you at the aspathre? No? My son has ear ache. I'll bring him to your house right away.'

Aspathre is a lingual variation of 'aspithal' or hospital.* There is no use explaining to patients that my aspathre is a one-room clinic.

Thus I began to see patients at home too. They would sometimes come in the early hours of the morning or late at night and I would have fobbed them off were it not for my tender-hearted husband. ('Just go and *see* what's wrong…') We partitioned off a portion of the veranda and I stocked up on some tablets, salves, injections, bandages and splints. Rural cordiality ensures that patients are willing to wait while I finish bathing, boiling the milk, burning chapatis or finishing a call. Some evenings I would return from my walk to find Vijay with half a dozen patients in our living room. An old woman coughing, a baby crying, a boy retching and my dear husband offering glasses of water, toys, reassuring words. The curious among them would get a conducted tour of the house, only to go away disappointed by the confusion of books and paper in every room. Some of the privileged classes are put off by the equalizer-effect of my scruffy clinic. 'You should discourage these labourers,' says a neighbour.

Why?

'They spread all sorts of diseases. And how can you trust them? They will observe everything, then come back and rob.'

Never mind that there has been no such incident in the village. The same neighbour cannot believe I encourage workers to send their children to school.

'If they study and land better jobs, where will we find workers during the coffee-picking season?' he asks.

The patients who seek treatment at home are the daily-wage earners—colourful, chatty, curious. They are neatly turned out unless they come straight from work. The fish-seller stops by

---

*'Hospital' is derived from 'hospice' which is derived from 'hospes' in Latin. It is where you go when you are sick. The words host and hospitality pertain to guests and hosts. Hostility and hostage are sibling words.

late in the evening. He has had no time to go home for a bath before coming to the clinic and is apologetic about the odours he brings with him. A woman who I am treating for her arthritic pains regularly requests me to 'hide' a few hundred rupees for her, safe from her husband. I think the man knows, or do I imagine the frown on his face when he meets me?

Excitement is always round the corner. Patients come in with the warning signals of a 'heart attack', with epileptic seizures, dog bites and injuries following drunken brawls. One early afternoon there came the grumble of an agitated motorbike approaching our house. It signalled an emergency of some sort. The bike bumped to a halt in our front yard, inches away from our semi-sacred tulsi plant so lovingly protected by bricks. Rajan, who was riding the bike, sprang away as it fell over. Mani the pillion-rider jumped too, but landed in a sprawl next to the spinning wheels, entangled in which was an incredibly long yellowish-brown snake, heaving and whipping at the metal spokes that imprisoned it. Rajan had a bite on his shin, and Mani was in shock which changed to relief when he realized that the snake was not a cobra, krait or viper. 'It's a rat snake,' he said, backing away nevertheless. Mani is a carpenter and in constant demand for his work. Rajan, a self-taught plumber, can be counted on to resolve all pipeline dilemmas. They had picked up the unfortunate passenger when negotiating a stretch of coffee plantation in order to take a shorter route into town. The bite of a rat snake causes a severe chemical reaction. Rajan would need treatment for a month, or perhaps two if the bite got infected but he would recover. For the snake, it was the last journey.

Snake, wasp and scorpion bites used to be more common in Kodagu, a predominantly agricultural district. Now many of the plantation workers use footwear and are better protected. Tribal culture keeps people close to nature. We have always depended on the animal and plant world for sustenance. The butcher used to wrap the purchase in a plantain leaf and tie it with a string stripped from its fibrous rib. Leaves of turmeric and plantain were used to wrap food or tacked together into shallow bowls in which just-plucked blooms were kept fresh by flower-sellers.

My sister's husband has fascinating stories about his great grandfather who was a doctor in Madikeri in the years before independence. Kongetira Mandanna was a Licensed Medical Practitioner who compounded his own medicines in his dispensary. As a young boy, my brother-in-law would watch him measure, sieve and weigh various chemicals with magical-sounding names—belladona, phosphorica, bismuth, gentian violet, terp vasaka. These the doctor would grind into powders and pastes or titrate and distil to make syrups and lotions, muttering words like, emollient, demulcent, astringent, emetic and carminative as he went about his work. He dispensed tinctures, elixirs and digestives, salves and powders in individually wrapped bits of paper on which he wrote the dosage. Dr Mandanna's precious possessions were his stethoscope with its fat rubber tubing, his satchel in which he carried the oft-needed medicines and his well-thumbed, heavily underlined, bound and rebound copy of the British Pharmacopoeia.

Sitting in my clinic with its electric light, the chemist's shop nearby and a laboratory in the same building, I think about the professional life of such a doctor in the days gone by. He would see patients in his own home and also make home visits. He would walk, or ride in a bullock-cart or on horseback. If a rich family needed his services they might send a box-carriage. He would risk his safety at night to see a child with fever and delirium, an elderly man who had suffered a stroke or a young woman in the pangs of a difficult childbirth. It was not uncommon for a doctor to spend an entire night or even several days in a sick person's home, administering medicines, applying a poultice, bandaging wounds, lancing boils and sewing up wounds.

As doctors, we learn every day from our patients. I see ten to fifteen patients in a day. A good number of them read like the pages of a medical textbook. I am about to prescribe a cough-suppressing medicine to a middle-aged woman with a persistent cough when she says, 'Never had it so bad. It wakes me every night and I have to sit up…' I put down my pen and reach for my stethoscope. 'Let me check you once more.' Yes, the lungs were speaking—the papery scratch of inhalation, the fine crackle in the base of the lungs is unmistakable. I cross out the prescription for a cough syrup and give her a small dose of a diuretic to stimulate the kidneys and rewrite her blood pressure medication. A few weeks later, she returns to say her cough has disappeared and she can breathe a lot better. Her cough was the sign of a failing heart. The pumping action had been weakened, blood was damming back in the veins and seeping fluid into the lungs. I nearly missed it.

That same day I see two cases of skin disease, a woman with a lump in the breast, one with intestinal tuberculosis, a young man with recalcitrant fits, a couple with marital problems, a nineteen-year-old welder with giddiness, an alcoholic with terminal liver failure. They need more time than the few minutes I need for a patient with a minor ailment like throat infection or a stomach upset. The epileptic will need a readjustment of his medicines; skin lesions are better seen under proper sunlight so I step out with the patient for a better look. The woman with tuberculosis will need blood tests; the young man with giddiness should not be working in the printing press with its noisy, old-fashioned printing machine. And I must stir up my grey matter to help solve a very tricky marital discord. There is reading to be done, and the pulling out of memory cards from my brain: a daily exercise in self-styled medical education.

A pleasant-mannered young man has been visiting my clinic for some time now. He comes with one or the other of his ageing parents. The very first time when I had finished examining his father, he asked: 'Could you please explain how exactly this thing called prostate is troubling him?'

My desk is littered with scraps of paper for scribbling dietary details and drawing diagrams to illustrate what happens in a disease; or how a surgery can overcome the problem. Patients are hardly ever curious about their own bodies. It is so much easier to put the responsibility of illness on the doctor, to take the prescription and get out quick. What patients do ask is the size of the scar after a surgery, the number of stitches, the duration of the hospital stay. To this young man who asked me about his father's prostate, I explained with a diagram the mechanism by which the prostate when enlarged blocks the flow of urine, and the different modes of treatment. His father opted for a course of medicines. The next time the young man brought his mother, a diabetic with gall stones. When I had examined her, he placed a notebook before me. 'I'd be grateful if you could kindly—' I explained, with a diagram. The mother said, 'No surgery please. The stones are not much trouble. I'll keep them for now.' Noting down a few points about her diet in the notebook I saw that the son had pasted the diagram I had drawn of an enlarged prostate inside the notebook.

To be well-informed about one's illness is the first step to healing; to be alert to mis-information is just as essential.

23

The Four Prongs of Illness

'My scientific studies have afforded me great gratification; and I am convinced that it will not belong before the whole world acknowledges the results of my work.'—Gregor Mendel, the father of modern genetics

Between birth and death, the body is the only place of shelter that we have. In the spring and summer years of life, we rarely think of the physical body except in terms of 'appearance'. The mirror is the sole influencer of the many decisions we make regarding this, while ignoring the ever-busy, complex factories within. With age, as attrition sets in and complaints from various parts of the body begin to overwhelm, we realize that the body is so much more than a carapace. There is more time, and more reason to be kind to our aging physicality. But alas, if we have not learnt to understand it early on, it is impossible to develop an intimacy when it has begun to tire and fray; to weaken and wither. It is essential to understand the body, and to recognize why we fall ill. The most common underlying factors of illness are:

- Genetic or inherited factors
- Stress
- Nutrition
- The environment

Most ailments are caused by one, or a combination of the above and compounded by the lack of physical activity. Once you know how and why you got that skin rash or diabetes or sciatica or the breathlessness, you are only a step away from learning how to prevent it, or how to hasten the cure. It is strange then that when I try to explain the *why* of any illness, patients are perplexed. 'Is it not your job to set it right?' is their silent rebuke. Ah well. A great many of us could live to be a hundred and twenty or more, if we tried to know ourselves.

Ignorance of one's own illness is shockingly common. Patients are willing to undergo tests, swallow pills, suffer injections and spend a lot of money to retrieve health. But health is not a commodity purchased from the medical profession. By making an attempt to improve your Health IQ, you can be less dependent on doctors.

Ever wondered how genetics and stress cause disease?

Gregor Johann Mendel, an Augustinian monk in 19th-century Austria, was a lover of botany. Monasteries of the time excelled in scientific research and experiments and Mendel was encouraged to further his study in plant biology. He experimented on hybrid pea plants and discovered how certain traits in a parent are inherited by the offspring. His work became the basis of the study of genetics.

The discovery of the Deoxyribonucleic Acid or DNA (by Crick and Watson in 1954) as the basic unit of individual identity was central to the study of genetics. The gene is the essence of a living cell. The abnormality of certain genes when passed from parent to offspring cause genetic or inherited disease. Haemophilia is a classic example, a sort of celebrity among genetic disorders because it was found to be prevalent in certain royal families of Europe and it took many young imperial lives. Diabetes, asthma, mental illness and malignant disease are few of the other diseases which may be inherited. Research into the mechanism of inheritance of a disease has helped in better management of such illness. As mentioned before, you might want to encourage your child to marry outside your caste and religion for it will protect the health of your grandchildren.*

*

Stress is caused by high-pressure situations that give rise to anxiety and worry. Sustained or recurring stress can affect health. Migraine, hyperacidity, irritable bowel syndrome, asthma, mental illness, skin disorders and backache can be caused by stress, or exacerbated by it. Even in the (seemingly) tranquil rural setting where I work, stress is a constant factor, especially among the poor. Nothing is more worrisome than hunger, homelessness, unemployment and a lack of dignity. They increase stress levels to an alarming degree and can precipitate serious illness.

Do pardon me if I appear to trail off a little here. At the beginning of this chapter, I mentioned four prongs of illness plus the lack of physical activity as the main drivers of sickness. Of course there is one more factor and that is emotional equanimity or grace.

Our emotions affect our long-term well-being; and what is well-being if it merely consists of smoothly functioning body parts? I have long wrestled with the concept of emotional grace and tried to make sense of it. It provides us with the ability to understand and act towards the collective betterment of people everywhere, without the prejudice of narrow divisive factors. It is our ability to love (spouse, child, parent, family, country, community) *without* having to hate another's child, family, country or community. We should not need to have enemies to love what is perceived as ours, be it our country or our kith and

*DNA studies and correlation with disease patterns shows the advantage of inter-community and inter-racial marriage in reducing the incidence of serious illness in future generations. Nature has always known this, and shown this.

kin. Like nationalistic fervour: when it is defined by the need to hate another country and its people, it becomes second-rate—as you might have noticed.

The world is abuzz with negativity caused by divisions. It allows massacres, assassinations, bombings, beheadings, lynchings, 'honour' killings; and other utterly coarse and destructive notions which attempt to criticize and curtail the conduct of others while loving our own. Emotional grace and equanimity are seen in those who eschew such dangerously negative concepts and actions. Without this inner wellness, a smoothly polished outer shell is of little value.

So, never forgetting the need for this inner wellness, every one of us should try and understand the body, its functions and the causes of malfunction.

24

The Food We Eat

We live because of it, and at times for it, but we cannot live without it. So forgive me this rather long chapter which deals with human fodder.

Lucullus, the epicurean of ancient Rome, was once asked why he did not invite guests home to partake of his sumptuous dinners. Did he not care to overwhelm them with his showmanship while enjoying their company? His imperious reply: 'Lucullus dines with Lucullus.' Wisdom lies in knowing and appreciating the food we eat.*

Nearly half the world's population survives on less than the required amounts of food; the rest of us eat way too much. Indians, like Americans, serve outsized portions. In the Middle Eastern countries, deep-fried meats and snacks are favoured. We worry about the waistline but care little about wastage. Fat used to be a sign of wealth and prosperity until about a hundred years ago when it became clear that fat people are more prone to disease. Sixty per cent of the patients who visit my clinic are well on their way to weakened hearts, afflicted livers and the degeneration of other organs all brought on by ill-considered eating.

Diseases that were once the privilege of the upper-class now punish all of society. Nobody is spared. Ten years ago, the

*I am neither an epicurean nor wise, but one of the most pleasurable and wise books I have read on food is *The Art of Eating* by M.F.K. Fisher.

intensive-care units of hospitals catered to the moneyed class. It was they who presented with acute heart attack, diabetic coma or stroke. Now it is as common to see the poor labourer, the domestic worker, the lorry driver and clerk suffering from the same diseases. Worse, it is changing into a reverse trend, because awareness about quality food and regular exercise will always reach the educated first. A person moving from poverty to relative wealth goes for convenience foods and a ride in an autorickshaw instead of walking the distance or footing it to the bus stop. He is doing fine, he can buy biscuits and sweets for his kids, indulge the family with fried snacks and fizzy pleasures that were once a luxury.

The average life expectancy of sixty-eight years among Indians conceals a jaggedly wide range of life expectancies. To live for thirty-five to forty years is considered fortunate among many tribal communities hindered as they are by the scarcity of food and the addiction to alcohol. Small communities everywhere are at greater risk of extinction because hereditary diseases are compounded by marriage within a small circle. The Muslims in southern India, once constitutionally strong, have allowed their health to be undermined by unwise eating habits and an absolute abhorrence of vegetables. Many of the educated, fifty-plus generation ate much better food when young than we do now. Tinned, bottled and packet foods were a rarity reserved for special occasions, so we did not consume too much of chemical preservatives, stale oil and the infamous maida* that go into such foods. Grains were eaten whole or powdered in small mills, thus retaining the husk which is high in fibre

---

*Maida is finely-milled wheat powder with the husk removed, thus denuding it of all goodness and life. It was popularly known as 'American flour' or 'merkin powder'. I used to write down the shopping lists for my mother and when she wanted to make some fancy snack like kal-kals or cake, 'Merkin powder' was on the list. This gift from America now comes labelled as 'refined flour'. (But I think it should be renamed as 'defiled flour'.)

and minerals. Kodavas (numbering a little over a lakh) ate a nourishing diet of wild meat, fresh greens and mushrooms with rice used in a variety of steamed preparations.* It was common practice for young men to hunt in the jungles beyond the coffee plantations and return with a rabbit, a wild fowl or a brace of partridge. Pork—fire-roasted, fried, dried or pickled—was essential fare in every home; pork fat preserved in earthenware pots and hung in the kitchen came in handy for perking up some vegetable that might otherwise leave the table untouched.

When hunting became illegal, we had to make do with the meat and fish from the market.† Families cherished their chicken coops, pig-sties and cattle-sheds, and maybe a small pond, with fish and duck. One variety of fish, the size of a child's little finger, abounded in the marshy fields of paddy and eaten with rice rotis was a breakfast favourite. Sardines were brought by Mapla traders from coastal Kerala. They came early mornings with the freshly caught fish in large tins which they carried on their heads. A rupee for a hundred slithering sardines. The physical demands of life in the rugged terrains of the hills combined with labour in the paddy fields demanded a high-protein diet, laced with a decent amount of fat for strength and muscle growth. Meat-eating rustics will not waste money on vegetables sold in the market, which they say is only water, and bad for the bones. Seasonal vegetables and fruit like mushroom, tender bamboo shoot, greens of a dozen varieties, yams, unripe banana and jackfruit are preferred.

---

*Coarsely powdered rice mixed with coconut and jackfruit, wrapped in banana leaf and steamed was the snack we ate when we came home from school. 'Fried food makes you fat and proud, steamed food makes you strong,' is a saying we grew up with.

†Poaching, and the eating of wild meat is by no means uncommon: Some months ago a young man who works in Bangalore and was back home in Kodagu for the weekend fell ill with an upset stomach. 'I ate porcupine meat for lunch yesterday,' he told me, casually.

My mother was operated for a broken hip when she was past ninety. 'If I did not know her age, I would have said she was seventy,' the surgeon said, so surprised he was by the healthy condition of her muscles and bone. She is closely matched by two of her sisters while their older brother died when he was just short of 102.

Kodavas are a hard drinking community. We worship our ancestors with meat and drink. Our grandmothers learned to make fermented wines with every fruit that grows here and we have a veritable range of spirits that have been distilled at home. Many a lady in her twilight years who comes to my clinic with a health disturbance will tell me about the 'little something' she takes every night. 'It helps me sleep.' My wholehearted approval is rewarded with a grateful smile. Keep going, madam. Only, don't let your granddaughters in medical school pour it out for you. I know of one who at times took a sip before ministering to her granny…

The rearing of farm animals and birds is on its way out, given that agricultural labour is migrating to the towns and cities. Meat and fish are bought from the butchers or in their processed or frozen form. In many homes in the villages of Kodagu you will still see chickens—rust brown, orange, stippled, multihued or deep black. If means allow, there are a few grunting pigs, and cows. Milk that is freshly sourced is freely available in our village, and will be for a few more years.

In the 1850s the British introduced the growing of coffee in Kodagu. Lush fields of paddy, once the visual delight of the post-monsoon months and the very backbone of our lives, were sacrificed in favour of the more lucrative cash-crop. With the use of fertilizers and pesticides on thousands of hectares of land, the soil began to lose its natural defences. Fruit trees perished. Modernity brought many conveniences, including motor vehicles, television, packaged foods and sedentary habits and ill health.

Kodagu is only a tiny district but the change in lifestyle and environment is not unique. Most of India has enjoyed prosperity with initiatives which have later proved to be unwise. It is also not entirely true that nutritional wisdom comes only from our ancestors. Tradition demands a certain fixity, at times stubborn, to age-old customs. Feasting, according to many traditions, is about gluttony; the gorging on food and drink. Mutton biryani, beef curry, Christmas cake, deep-fried snacks and alcohol in excess, with the end result of heartburn or an ache in the heart of a more serious variety. There is as much foolishness as wisdom in traditional knowledge. Milk is widely believed to cause the formation of pus in the body and try as you might, you cannot get patients to take it in any form until he or she has recovered from an illness or surgery. Milk is known to aggravate chest and nasal congestion in those who suffer from milk intolerance but it is not universal. In Bihar they swear by the blood-enriching qualities of baidana ka ras or pomegranate juice, which is rich in vitamins and minerals and patients are known to survive on nothing but this for days on end. While fasting for short periods is good for the well-fed, it can be disastrous in those who are in urgent need of nutrition. The fruit carts that routinely sell fruit outside every hospital gate are never short of apples, the most sought-after fruit for the sick. They glow with wax polish which ensures longevity (of the fruit, not the consumer). It must make a week-long journey by truck to reach your fruit-seller in Trichy or Kottayam and is thus depleted of many of its nutrients. Tomatoes and curds are given up for most of the year for fear of causing chest infections.*

---

*Miraculously, this easily perishable vegetable has developed the peculiar trait of staying firm and fresh forever. I left half a dozen tomatoes on an open rack in the kitchen, in March, our hottest month. The tomatoes remained firm for all of four weeks. Not even a wrinkle. Frustrated, I used them up. They were quite tasteless but unperished.

Rice is 'the staff of life' in southern India. With vegetables, pulses, milk and curds as additional foods, we are well propped. The spices used in sambar, kootan, avial and moru kolambu and a host of vegetarian dishes bewildered the British colonials so much, they quickly coined the word curry to describe the lot. Sattu, made of roasted and powdered channa dal, is the popular energizer of all true Biharis. It was my health drink when we lived in Mokama. Daliya, the porridge made with broken wheat, is favoured in the northern states while the delicious poha of Maharashtra (or avalakki in Karnataka) is superior in nutrition to the expensive breakfast flakes. The Tamils love their kanji, Kannadigas their ragi mudde and Malayalis swear by steamed puttu and bananas.

While at least 40 per cent of Indians say they are vegetarian, many among them are occasional or surreptitious meat-eaters. Along with 'social drinking', the eating of chicken curry or mutton biryani is an upwardly mobile social activity, be it at home, hotel or a shanty-town bar. Meat-eating is a weekly ritual in families with modest means and beef and fish are clear favourites, after chicken. The 'vegetarian' meat-eaters love chicken, perhaps because of its blandness and ease of preparation. Sadly, the meat comes from birds reared in large chicken factories where the chick is processed as soon as it is hatched. It is readied for the market, injected with hormones and antibiotics which fatten them quickly, so the transition from chick to chicken happens in a few weeks. The outcome? Frequent bouts of severe dyspepsia and serious antibiotic resistance in chickens.

Additionally, the banning of beef in many parts of the country has hit those of us who have a preference for this excellent form of lean meat which is also the most nutritive and least expensive. But the four letter B word has become incendiary and somehow 'anti-national' so I will not waste space to tell you about its many values, its richness in iron and

Vitamin B12, its hearty deliciousness and the goodness of its protein content, so vital for growth and strength. The price of pulses has doubled; milk-products are not cheap. In some states, eggs are not allowed in mid-day school meals because they will upset the sentiments of vegetarian students. In modern India, it is wise to remember that sentiment matters more than health.

I try to convince my patients to pay attention to the food they eat but few care to listen. One woman whose son has a poor appetite and rotting teeth refuses to believe that giving him a packet of biscuits first thing every morning is foolish. After hearing me out about the evils of packeted junk, she declared, 'My son would rather starve than eat home food.' His taste buds have been dulled by the sugary drinks, fried snacks, toffees, crisps and biscuits and noodles. 'By God's grace we earn much more now, between my husband and myself we bring home about 20,000 a month. We can afford to let him eat what he likes.'

The director of a company that makes a popular brand of milk biscuits recently said in an interview that mothers are 'aware' of the health benefits of glucose biscuits;* that it is the first solid food given to babies when they are weaned off mother's milk. The power of advertising! Children who are encouraged to eat biscuits for breakfast are known to continue with this habit even when they are in high school. A young woman who works as a help in the house of a friend told her,

---

*Biscuits are sold under so many eye-catching names and ingredients which tempt you to reach for a packet: milk biscuits, digestives, sugar-free, chocolate-flavoured, vitamin-enriched and the rest. I was a fan of biscuits for a very long time, so I know them all. Except for a small niche of biscuit makers who use organic whole grains, healthy oils and jaggery, the rest are mostly made of maida or refined flour, unhealthy fats, salt and loads of sugar. While I don't exactly belong to the ban-the-biscuit brigade, I do think it should only be eaten as an occasional snack. The same goes for all bakery items. Bakers need not despair. If they want to stay in business, they must quickly switch to healthy alternatives.

with great pride, that she never cooks breakfast. Her family of four starts the day with tea and a packet each of glucose biscuits and only her husband's mother eats the rice left over from the previous day. India will definitely need more dentists to take care of a generation with early dental caries.

I am not yet done on this subject, sorry. The media supplies a great deal of misinformation in the form of advertisements tangled with facts, resulting in foolish beliefs such as the one that holds that biscuits and 'health drinks' are brain food. Half an hour of watching television can turn your brain into a puddle of greed. Unhealthy high-end pap gets shamelessly lauded by celebrities who will not touch them. The more expensive the goods being sold, the more treacherously untrue the superlative qualities extolled.

Unethical advertising is nothing recent. When Coca Cola entered the Indian market in the early sixties, school students in Delhi were treated to free bottles of the iced drink, a fancy metal ruler painted white and a twenty-minute film about the magic drink. To hang out with friends over iced cola and potato wafers was the fashionable past-time for any teenager. The flavoured and coloured sugar water plus carbon dioxide and some caffeine became the favourite of generations, quietly adding to the burden of diabetes, hypertension and other metabolic diseases besides dental caries.

A few years ago when a company producing a popular brand of noodles was accused of supplying stuff that contained toxic ingredients, it was taken off the shelves. Hundreds of food products with similar toxic substances are sold and eaten every day. Snacks, breads, biscuits and cakes that we purchase from bakeries and confectioners are made of maida, or processed tapioca, both being devoid of any nutrition barring the starch that converts to sugar inside our bodies. Packaged foods contain large amounts of unhealthy fats, preservatives and taste enhancers. Meanwhile the noodles are back on the shelves and a certain shrewd businessman has taken over a major portion of the entire snack industry by claiming to be an authentic, Hinduized version and therefore blameless.

I saved up the following anecdote to end this chapter with.

Soon after the uprising in 1857 against British occupation, we got our first three universities. The rulers understood the need for the better education of natives, particularly in English, so they could administer the vast country with the help of these educated Indians who could manage clerical and other sub-ordinate jobs. The learning of English became easier and more regulated, opening windows to the writings of Western thinkers. Those with the means to a college education were thus enabled to compare local customs, prejudices and practice with those of the West. The next fifty or sixty years brought an era of remarkable change in Indian intellectual thought.

The following incident happened a decade or so after the first three universities of Madras, Bombay and Calcutta came to life. The Nizam of the princely state of Hyderabad suffered from an 'incurable' illness. The wisest among the siddhars, hakims, vaidyars, homoeopaths, praanic healers and swamis with special yogic powers were consulted. They came from far and stayed at the palace brewing their concoctions, chanting mantras, grinding metallic powders and animal bones in order to hit upon the cure for the mysterious royal ailment. His Highness lost weight, lost sleep, became listless and tired. When all else failed, he called for the English physician, Dr William Campbell McLean.

After careful questioning and examination, the physician said: 'Your Highness. I will be able to cure your malady.'

'Indeed?' said the Nizam, brightening. 'Don't ask me to take any of your foul firangi medicines though. I refuse.'

'All I want is that you follow my advice on what you eat and drink.'

The Nizam laughed. 'I eat the best and the reddest of meat

from goats specially fed and cared for. The meat is cooked in chicken or mutton fat. As for the sweets, they are always made with butter and ghee and virgin-white sugar. I drink choice sherbets and wines. There is no one in all of Asia who eats and drinks so well.'

'You will have to give up meat, eggs and all types of sweets for three months. And no sherbets or wines.'

'Hai, Allah! You mean I should starve?'

Dr McLean assured him that although the food would not feel so good on the tongue, it would certainly make him healthy once more. 'I might as well warn you that if you ignore your illness now, it may be too late…'

The Nizam had no choice. Instead of meats, wines and sweet sherbets, his table now boasted of steamed gourds, raw cabbage in vinegar, endless quantities of boiled beans, roasted dals, vegetable juices and dry chapatis that made him nauseated with disgust. So much so that he no longer visited the harem; the queens wrung their hands in frustration. The Nizam persisted with the harsh diet. Within weeks he began to feel better, slept one continuous sleep during the night and was feeling strong enough to ride his horse, although the joys of shikaar and the gluttonous feasts that followed were forbidden by the British doctor. In three months he was back to normal. Having effusively thanked and rewarded his healer, the Nizam said he was curious to know how the white man had nailed his illness and cured it when all others had failed.

'You said you were thirsty all the time and in spite of drinking jugs of water your tongue was dry,' answered Dr McLean. 'You needed a commode by your bed, remember? You used it dozens of times, day and night? They are the symptoms of diabetes, where the blood sugar shoots up. The epicurean delights enjoyed by your majesty were the chief offenders. I cured you with a diet that helped to bring the sugar levels down to normal.'

Impressed by the miracle cure of his diabetes by the allopathic physician, the Nizam decided to set up a medical college in the city. The Osmania Medical College was established in 1864 and the twelve students who enrolled in the very first batch were handpicked by the Nizam for their aptitude and intelligence.

25

The Environment

A dozen members of a family were gathered in the living room. Short-eats were served, tea drunk and I was making polite conversation with a dear old lady when these words drew my attention: '...it was like some fantasy, with bubbles floating everywhere. A man on a scooter looked like he had hurried out from his bath without washing off the soap, the girl sitting pillion was spitting bubbles and a little boy's head was wreathed in them.'

A niece was describing the morning scene on a busy road in Bangalore. It runs alongside a once-beautiful lake now ravaged by chemical and sewage effluents from factories. At certain times of the day, when the breeze is strong it churns up the foam on the lake which gets sprayed on the road, engulfing traffic in bubble and fizz. As I listened, a Sunday from my medical college days came to mind. I was going to a party in one of the houses that overlooked the lake. From college we took a bus which stopped close to the area. We lingered for a while near the lake to look at the pink lotuses on clear water, the small boats in the distance, the trees preening on the sky and in the clear waters of the lake, and a few couples having a morning to themselves. Today, that image sounds like fantasy.

Traffic congestion, poorly maintained vehicles, coal fires, wood smoke and factories are the foremost purveyors of polluted air. Three out of nine vehicles need to be hospitalized for geriatric care. They emit thick black clouds toxic fumes from their exhausts, thus disregarding anti-pollution laws. Asthma, lung cancer, heart disease and hormonal imbalance leading to infertility are aggravated by pollution. Traffic police, pedestrians and those dependent on public transport are more at risk while those inside air-conditioned cars get away. Or perhaps they do not. Long exposure to this conditioned air is itself damaging. Pollution will nab every one of us, sooner or later. The just-retired managing director of a company who lives in Delhi found himself behind a lorry once. As he was getting out of his Peugeot to meet someone across the road, a gush of black smoke blew in his face. The next thing he remembers is waking up in hospital, having vomited as he inhaled the smoke and then losing consciousness. The accidental breathing of poisonous gas damaged his lungs and left him permanently afflicted with a serious breathing problem. He is house-bound and needs oxygen to get through each day. One of the most popular car makers cheated the public for years, using computer chips that give false safety levels of pollutants produced by the car engines.

Back in the 1940s and '50s, smog caused an alarming increase of respiratory diseases in the very young and the elderly in London.* When laws came into force against polluting vehicles and factories, the smog lessened and so did chronic lung ailments which used to fill hospitals in the winter months. In the early 1970s, a paediatrician driving to work from his suburban home into London noticed large plots where vegetables like cabbage, squash, carrot and beetroot were grown adjacent to the motorways. Over the years he was able to correlate the high incidence of lead poisoning in children living

*The smog was so bad that the Greenwich Mean Time (GMT) Tower had to be shifted to another site in UK because of the dense screen of smog which prevented the proper functioning of apparatus.

in that area to the vegetables they ate. The vegetables were contaminated with lead which led to brain damage, impaired intelligence and poor learning abilities in the children. This set off a campaign against the use of lead in petrol, heated debates in Parliament and ultimately the compulsory use of unleaded petrol. Forty years on, in India we are no way near cleaning up our act, and we have ended up panting harder than ever before.

For two months towards the end of 2016, Vijay and I stayed in a modest locality in Bangalore. Shops and homes spilled on to the narrow streets congested with traffic. Every empty lot in every street was used to chuck garbage. Dogs, cows, buffaloes, rodents the size of big cats, crows and the very poor scavenged in the rubbish. A large municipal truck with Swachch Bharat emblazoned on its flanks came three days a week to collect garbage with which it lumbered on, filth dripping off, while two-wheelers, cars, school buses and pedestrians moved alongside. Some of the biggest and purportedly the best of hospitals were a ten-minute drive away; shops, slums, mansions, vendors and families live next to these volcanoes of disease.

And yet we are puzzled if visitors to our country label us a filthy people. When a writer says that India is 'a land of two thousand stinks' I feel my nation is being slighted. The truth is that our senses are so deadened, we no longer smell what others smell. We revere the family, we revere the home, we believe these spaces to be sacred and we have them cleaned—by our servants whom we pay poorly—again and again. We clean our bodies repeatedly, we sanitize our houses while ignoring the muck piling up outside our gates.

Literacy does not always change such habits but it helps.* Take Pune. Until 2006, several hundred metric tonnes of waste from the city of Pune were being dumped at a garbage

---

*Sikkim, with an 81 per cent literacy rate, is listed as the cleanest state in India, followed by Kerala and Mizoram, which have higher literacy rates of 94 and 91 per cent respectively.

site in nearby Pimpri-Chichwad. As this area became more industrialized and new housing colonies sprang up, the local municipality closed its doors to the Pune waste. Thereafter a quick decision was taken by the Pune Municipal Corporation (PMC) to divert its waste to dumping sites in two nearby villages, Phursingi and Urali Devachi. A few months after this insult was hurled at them, the villagers rebelled. They denied entry to the garbage-laden trucks. The PMC pleaded and using various pressure-tactics, managed to continue dumping for another year, with the assurance of setting up a system to segregate and recycle waste.

The year went by, followed by a grace period of three and then six months and then twelve. It was summer. A fire broke out in the garbage dump due to large amounts of methane gas produced from the waste from the intensely high temperatures within the mass of flammable debris. The fire brigade, using twenty fire engines, struggled for ten days to douse the fire. The rag-pickers who survive on material picked from the dumps sustained burns on their feet as their cheap plastic chappals melted in the heat.

This time the villagers stepped up their protests and blocked all the vehicles from coming into their villages. Pune began to stink, stray dogs multiplied, and so did rodents, flies, mosquitoes and germs. People came out in large numbers to protest against the municipality, the government, the shop-owners, the greedy house-builders and the dirty rabble who lived uncleanly in slums. I wonder if any of the protestors felt that they too were blame-worthy. Pune was once a relatively clean city, a hub of education and intellectual progress, of literate women and social welfare. Some of our foremost national leaders emerged from the institution of learning in Pune; the military cantonment, the National Defence Academy and the Armed Forces Medical College furthered its glory. Along with Bangalore it is now a favoured feeding place of digital technology. But its frenzied growth in the last thirty years has reduced it into a quagmire of poor planning and congestion. Its garbage output is 1700 tonnes a day. Thanks to the villagers of Phursinghi and Urali Devachi, Pune was forced to initiate the segregation of waste, composting, recycling of plastics and the generation of fuel.

The PMC asked the central government for Rs 350 crores towards this initiative. The centre released Rs 87 crores, a bit too readily. Why 87 crores? Because it was the amount required to clean up the area near the airport where garbage sites increased 'bird activity' in the skies, endangering airplanes with bird-hits which can lead to accidents. The government saw the importance of preventing bird-hits to aircrafts. You cannot expect the government to see any importance in rag-pickers burning their hands and feet as a result of decomposing garbage, or dying from diseases spread by the handling of waste. I'm not cribbing about the 87 crores, I'm just startled by the irony of it.

Undisposed-of waste leads to indisposed humans. (Twenty-two of the thirty most polluted cities in the world are in India, with Ghaziabad being in second place, after Hotan in China.) Visitors from the cities go into raptures about the clean air in our villages. This clean-ness is not real, if you consider that our hinterlands are thinly populated in comparison to cities. Look closely and find out how waste is taken care of in our rural havens: most homes burn waste in their backyards, or if they do not have a backyard, it ends up by the roadside or in the nearest drain. There is no functioning alternative for the disposal of waste. Refuse of all types—from our public places, shops and homes—finally reach garbage dumps, which are enormous pits in the outskirts of rural villages and towns. Refuse: an aptly descriptive word for that which we cry-off as not ours once past it is past usefulness.

26

Can Your Job Kill You?

A boy of sixteen visits my clinic frequently with severe attacks of wheezing and bronchitis. He is the eldest of four, with a 'single' mother who works as a cook in a small eatery. Vidyut's breathing problems began two years ago when he dropped out of school to work in a shop selling chickens. He slaughters the birds—about thirty to forty of them every day. The mother refused to believe that the job was endangering his life until six months later when he had to be admitted to hospital for treatment. He now works in a bakery. Fortunately, he did not opt to work in a flour mill where the micro-fine dust raised by the milling of grains would be as dangerous as the flurry feathers, dust and dried faecal matter in a slaughterhouse for birds.

Over 40,000 Indians are reported to be dying every year from reasons related to their jobs. The figure only looks at registered workers who constitute barely 10 per cent of our workforce.*

Health hazards at work are so commonplace, we don't even notice. Traffic inspectors suffer chest ailments from daily

*Of the 264 million workers in India, only 26 million are in the organized sector. The regulatory authority that monitors occupational hazards for the entire country consists of 1,400 safety officers, 1,154 factory inspectors, and twenty-seven medical inspectors, making it practically impossible for them to make any impact. As for laws against unsafe working conditions, a mere 20 million workers are covered by laws that govern occupational safety.

exposure to vehicular fumes, backache from long hours of standing and the constant danger of being involved in an accident. This is collateral damage: the Bush Principle, if you recall. Construction workers develop lung disease from the inhalation of dust and paint fumes; deafness from the high-decibel sound of drills and machinery; and injuries caused by falling from a height. Workers in asbestos and granite industries handle toxic material with no protective gear and no awareness of the hazards involved. Women working in garment and textile industries must meet impossible targets of making 100 to120 garments an hour, with virtually no breaks in between. The cotton fluff that they breathe at work leads to chronic lung conditions that make them more susceptible to tuberculosis.

Perhaps the longest word in the English language is Pneumonoultramicroscopicsilicovolcanoconiosis, better known as silicosis. Of the one crore workers who toil in order to supply stone, cement and bricks for building our homes, shops and malls, many die early from the crippling effects of silicon dust which damages the delicate components of the lungs and interfere with oxygenation. The symptoms are easily mistaken for tuberculosis and followed by years of fruitless treatment when the only thing that can help is a change of profession. There are entire villages in a district in Telangana known as 'widows' villages' where the men work as stone-crushers, and die early from silicosis. The slate-pencil industry in Mandasaur reports a 59 per cent prevalence of the disease. There are lesser-known ways in which inhalation of fine particles can lead to life-threatening lung disease. It is now an established fact that wood smoke, so commonly used for cooking in villages, is responsible for a number of widely prevalent diseases like hypertension, ischaemic heart disease, diabetes and stroke. It can also lead to the same diseases afflicting unborn babies. If a pregnant woman inhales wood smoke while cooking, her newborn is at a higher risk for cardiac disease, diabetes and infertility. In the

Little Rann of Kutch in Gujarat many thousands of salt-pan workers acquire severe forms of skin disease due to the long-term contact with brine.

Rag-pickers who handle contaminated refuse, broken glass and inflammatory substances, and the sanitation workers who clean toilets, drains and sewers are the worst hit by their occupations. The occupational hazards of dealing with waste are multiple and largely undocumented. They endure the indignity of a job that no one else will do; they risk skin, lung and stomach infections and suffocation from noxious fumes when they plunge bare-bodied into clogged drains and manholes. Rag-pickers and those who clean sewers are prone to a host of diseases because of the work they must do. About 2000 sewer cleaners in our country die every year while cleaning septic tanks and manholes. This figure does not take into account the several thousands who die from close contact with waste. The life expectancy of these safai karmacharis (cleanliness workers) is at least twenty or thirty years below the national average of sixty-eight years. Not one of these brave warriors of filth have had a medal for courage pinned to their chests, not one of them gets a salute when his young body is carried away (sans the national flag to decorate it) for the last rites.

Take a look at the country as a whole: improper waste management and public disregard of sanitation is terrorism at work in broad daylight. We are a hundred times more likely to die from the deadly effects of toxins released from garbage than from the hands of a crazy gunman. We know it. We feel anger, disgust and outrage about this problem, which, by the way, is our own refuse. But we do nothing about it. We do not insist our government address the problem. We do not ask if a political candidate has a solution or even has waste management and cleanliness on his agenda. We prefer to think of an enemy as a man with a gun and a mission. That's easier than saying: I am part of the problem because of the refuse I generate.

The e-waste or the waste from electronic gadgets is quietly eating into the health of future generations. To add to this, we are the recipients of e-waste from several Western nations who pay to dump poisons in our territory. The 'clean rooms' of the high-tech electronics industry use several toxic chemicals. There is also the matter of the health of the workers in this sector. There are the call-centre workers who spend long hours at the computer and telephone. Their work is repetitive and intensive, with unrealistically high targets and constant surveillance. Most of these young men and women suffer from sleep deprivation, migraine, neck and back pain, eye strain and depression. The medical reasons are all too obvious.

Indian laws on occupational safety clearly state that it is the duty of the employer to ensure a safe working environment for employees. This applies to the organized sector, which is a mere 10 per cent of the total workforce. The rest, who work in the informal sector, do so without any safeguards or health benefits.*

Occupational safety is not high on the list of priorities with the trade unions in India. The unions believe it is more urgent to ensure employment and fair wages. It is easy enough to understand this: food and shelter first, and then everything else. Workers too, in their urgent desire to earn, are casual about the dangers. Whose responsibility is it, then, to ensure the safety of workers who make it possible for the rest of us to live in comfort? 'Millions of Indians have their lifespan shortened by decades, because of their occupation,' says Dr Bobby Joseph who heads the Department of Community Medicine and

---

*ESIS or Employees Social Insurance Scheme works as a social security and insurance scheme established by the Jawaharlal Nehru government in 1952. Its welfare facilities are available to small-scale industries with more than ten workers. The employee contributes1.5 per cent of her wages while the employer contributes 4.5 per cent. Thanks to the bureaucratic hurdles which come in the way, ESIS is less than satisfactory and does not cater to all who deserve it.

Occupational Health at St John's Medical College. 'Hazards at work undermine the nation's health. If we can feel proud about some of our medical achievements, we should also be ashamed of our indifference towards our workers.'

So what is the answer? 'Taking genuine steps to safeguard the workers is not really difficult, but it costs money. Most business ventures look to making money, not losing it.' He says there are companies which do more than others for occupational safety, but they are few. Most employers are as guilty as the government.

27

The SFL Triangle

'A night with Venus and a lifetime with Mercury.'—An early saying about syphilis

For the medical student, learning about the regions of the body where 'procreation flares' is an unremarkable experience. The details about organs are prosaic when compared to the thrills of sex experienced in novels and movies, and (maybe) a whiff of it in real life. However, it is easier to develop a dispassionate understanding of sex-related clinical situations when sex is neither the prima donna nor the prime accused. The whole point of having these organs is to propagate the species. This primal urge embodied in sexuality is the driving force of life as well as death.

The organs hide in a dark and private place and weigh no more than 250 grams when quiescent. Specific hormones control sexuality and the secondary features that make us male, female or transgendered. The hormones provide men with gruff voices and facial hair; they cause breast enlargement in women and give each gender certain body shapes. The deeper emotional differences pulse through life in alarming ways, challenging our ability to connect with each other, and leading to tensions that are uniquely…unique.

Of the many sexual diseases which beset mortals, venereal disease or sexually transmitted diseases (VD or STD) are the gravest, with syphilis being the most venerable, and the most feared (until the less exotic AIDS claimed the pedestal some forty years ago).

Syphilis was democratic: striking royals and rag-pickers alike. First described among soldiers in Italy in the 15th century, it was believed to have come from French soldiers who in turn blamed Egyptian prostitutes as the gift-bearers. Venereal diseases of all types are commonly the result of promiscuity, or having sex with multiple partners. The visha-kanyas or the poison-women of myth were perhaps thus afflicted. In the 15th century, the Italian physician and poet Girolamo Fracastoro wrote a three-volume epic poem on syphilis, from which the disease got its name and which I hope to read sometime.

Early treatment of syphilis with strong brews made from the bark of certain trees gave way to potions containing lead and mercury. As the pain and suffering were intense, newer drugs were tried. But their side-effects were often as dreadful as the disease.* There was no permanent cure until penicillin was discovered towards the end of World War II. By the late sixties, the disease had become uncommon enough to be exotic. As students we did see a few fresh cases, though: the typical painless ulcer on the penis which appears a few days after a sexual transgression and recorded in the patient's file as 'exposure: positive'. Fact couched in medical courtesy. The disease was confirmed through blood tests and clinical findings and treated with penicillin injections. Men carrying the secret guilt of an 'exposure' would come with imagined or real symptoms and ask for the injection. Mere reassurance was futile, for they went elsewhere, and since penicillin was effective against many other

*During World War I, soldiers afflicted by the disease were left to anoint each other with an unguent of mercury to ease the pain.

forms of venereal disease, doctors obliged. Syphilis causes fewer symptoms in women and is often undetected for years. Thus a young woman might unknowingly pass it on to her partner or her newborn.

Untreated syphilis can progress to the second, and the third stages affecting skin, bone, brain and other tissues. It hides behind a range of symptoms like soft swellings, an unsteady gait, poor dexterity, shooting pains in the legs, delusions, mental confusion or seizures. Before the detective medical eye discovered the offending organism under the microscope—the corkscrew-shaped *Treponema Pallidum*—the bizarre symptoms which brought a patient to hospital with late-stage syphilis were clubbed under a condition called the General Paralysis of the Insane (GPI). These symptoms included Romberg's sign (the inability to maintain balance with both arms raised and eyes shut), the lack of hand-eye coordination (like the inability to bring finger to nose in quick repetition), the Argyll Robertson pupils (abnormal and unequal size of pupils) and gumma (soft swellings which cause deformities) are some of the late signs of the disease. The patient could be an avuncular neighbour or the affectionate grandfather. Our neurology professor saw to it that we students got enough time to learn about the disease and therefore such treasures stayed in hospital for weeks, happily surprised with all the attention they received. One of our priced patients was a seventy-five-year-old who had a shoebox full of the carbon copies of the letters he had written to the Queen of England, demanding that she pay him hundred pounds, fifteen shillings and nine pence in return for the gold amulet owned by his father who lost his life in World War I. The said amulet was apparently snatched by her *soldiers*. He had written twelve letters to the queen and keenly awaited her reply. In older times, emperors in many parts of the world lived in happy mental confusion or in a state of total madness and delusional behaviour, and maybe with seizures, all of which could have been caused by the corkscrew germ. Think of all the madmen of history who ruled various corners of the planet, think about the eccentricities of kings and queens. How many had GPI?

World War I had resulted in a huge number of US soldiers coming back with the 'clap', a slang for venereal disease of which syphilis was the most eccentric in terms of the devilry it wreaked on its victim. What is far more outlandish and frankly criminal is this: in 1932, the Tuskegee Institute, in Alabama, in partnership with the US Public Health Service conducted trials on hundreds of syphilitics. *Treatment was withheld for these patients so that the natural progression of the disease could be scrutinized.* The study began eight years before the discovery of penicillin. But even after penicillin was proved to cure syphilis, it was not given to those being experimented upon in the clinical trial in Tuskegee. The majority of the human guinea pigs were Blacks who had no idea that treatment had been denied to them.*

The unethical nature of these dastardly experiments on syphilitics in Tuskegee began to be raised in the 1960s, that is, a full thirty years later when many sufferers had died of the untreated disease. Even then, it was decided that the study would continue until all the patients had died. Most of these 'under-trials' were likely to have been in their twenties when they got infected. In 1972 the news was leaked to the mainstream press

*It is significant that in Germany, Hitler had just begun his own human experiments whereby women with bodily or mental defects were sterilized against their will, in order to produce a superior, more perfect race. This concept of eugenics, first propounded by Galton in England, became popular among a small group of scientists in the US in the decade preceding World War II. Hitler got his idea by reading about it in a book by Alfred Ploetz (1860-1940), who was one of its votaries in the US. Hitler's subsequent descent towards the use of euthanasia for infants born with defects and then the mass killings of Jews and all the inconvenient 'criminal-minded, unwanted members of society' was connected to the initial concept of eugenics. Scientists who strongly opposed this form of Junk Science left Germany in large numbers. Where did most of them land up? In the US.

and therefore the study was hastily brought to a close. A court case followed and compensation was given to those who had escaped death from untreated syphilis. When Bill Clinton was president, the few surviving victims of the Tuskegee experiment were invited to the White House and offered a formal apology.

The US government obviously thought nothing of such acts because, in 1948, a US-sponsored experiment began in Guatemala which was even more brutal. Prisoners, soldiers and mental patients were artificially infected with the syphilitic germ without their knowledge and a study similar to the Tuskegee experiment was begun. I could not find out when it was stopped but again, a formal apology was made by the US government in 2010.*

Following the efficacy of penicillin, used extensively to cure patients during World War II, syphilis was silenced; a few decades later it resurfaced with the surge of HIV infections. Heterosexual habits, multiple partners and a lowered immunity makes HIV-infected persons more susceptible to syphilis. In 1999, 1.2 crore people worldwide were infected with syphilis and about a tenth of them died within a decade. Such lessons from history are not to be ignored. Besides, the spirochete's time may not be over yet.

*

The instinct that ensures procreation finds expression in an urgent desire to fit a certain part of one's body with certain part of another. It is fundamentally a body function like the urge to pee or defecate, but a gratification so compelling that it willingly breaks every custom, canon or directive that society might impose. Judging from advertisements that beckon from

*The difference between this and the initial brutalities of Hitler's regime seems to be this: the US was sly and discreet with such dastardly medical crimes; good sense came to the fore, eventually, and such experiments were stopped. Hitler's men were boastful and allowed the news to catch fire.

internet sites, news magazines and writings-on-the-walls that you try to or try not to look at, we have sexologists, perverts, venereologists, psychiatrists, counsellors and godmen ready with advice and therapy.

Sexually transmitted diseases are not always the result of a morally reprehensible act. They are passed on to innocent partners, newborn babies, and through contaminated needles. The social stigma for the sufferer is huge. Parents throw out children, wives forsake husbands, sons disown fathers and fathers disown sons.

Four years ago, a middle-aged man was admitted to our wards for terminal care of venereal disease, with complications, one of which was the severe narrowing of his urinary passage. It required mechanical stretching with metal dilators at regular intervals. He also had AIDS which was slowly consuming his body. His sons had witnessed his brutalities towards their mother from their childhood years. One day they returned from school to find her dead, her head crushed with a stone. The previous night, their father had beaten her senseless after a quarrel. Both boys left home once they were old enough, and never looked back. I remember the horror of loneliness in the eyes of this patient who knew he was dying and had no one who cared.

Moral indignation and the fear of sexually transmitted disease result in punishing the victim with human barbarity. Some years ago a Tamil youth suspected to have AIDS was set on fire in his own village. There have been a few more such incidents where the mob decides and enforces the penalty. There are hospitals which will not treat HIV-infected persons, citing the risk to other patients, although precautions which will ensure safety are simple and easy to follow.

Guilt related to sex often springs from an underlying reservoir of pain and sorrow. In rural communities, the doctor is also the counsellor. Sex, family and love form a triangle from which you can dredge so many stories of human uplift and misery. I call it the sfl triangle. (In small letters, in deference to its secretive personality where a doctor's discretion and confidentiality are paramount.)

A senior nurse once sought my help in a personal matter concerning her teenage daughter. The girl had become unduly rebellious, and hostile towards her mother. I knew her to be a well-mannered and pleasant teenager but I barely spoke to her except when she came to my clinic to offer sweets on her birthday or came home to borrow a book. The nurse's husband worked in another district and was home for a day on weekends. When I got to see the daughter alone she told me that she was waiting for the day when she could live in a hostel, away from her parents. Her mother was too controlling and possessive and except for school, did not let her out of sight. The girl was not allowed to speak to any boy, even a cousin or one of the teenagers on the hospital campus. She could visit the homes of their neighbours, but only with her mother.

Why the control, the exacting rules about boys at an age when every adolescent needs friends, I asked the nurse. Slowly and hesitantly the nurse told me how as a girl of ten she had been 'visited' by two uncles who used her until she got married. She confided in her husband soon after marriage and it caused a problem between them. Although he did not say it, he believed that she was to blame in some way for what those uncles did to her.

'I wish I wasn't married,' she said, her eyes filling with tears. 'I hate sex. It is far too painful. It is easier to let my husband go where he likes than subject myself to it. I don't want any such thing to happen to my daughter.' She constantly warned the girl about the dangers of mixing with boys, and the pain and the pitfalls of sex. She sincerely hoped that this only child of theirs would become a nun and be protected forever.

The following year the girl went to a boarding school and

everything seemed to be okay for a year. One day she asked to speak to me. 'I want to know if there is some reason for my dreams,' she blurted. 'They are always about my finding myself suddenly naked. Sometimes half-naked, sometimes fully so, in front of people. At times, I am in the bath or in toilet when someone opens the door…' She woke from her dreams with an overwhelming sense of shame and guilt. 'What am I to do about it? I've stopped talking to boys. I can't say why…but I'm afraid.' The mother had passed on her trauma to her daughter; she had instilled in the young girl her own fears. The daughter who never wanted to be a nun was cheered when told that such escape modes were not of any value unless she really wanted to join a nunnery. As she developed confidence, her self-esteem improved and she was able to enjoy the company of boys. I met her a year after her marriage. 'I'm okay now,' she said, smiling happily. 'Those dreams haven't disappeared, but I'm okay.'

Men are no better off when it comes to imagined horrors concerning sex. In rural areas with its one-doctor-sees-all concept, it is doubly hard. The patient is young or youngish, neatly turned out, with styled hair and the strong smell of perfume or aftershave and the strain of too much thinking showing on his face. He starts by talking a great deal about his indigestion or giddiness or headache and then as a seeming afterthought adds that he suffers from extreme weakness, due to 'too much leakage'. As soon as he has told you about the weakness, he forgets those other complaints. All he needs is reassurance about a normal activity and maybe some vitamins to make his visit seem worthwhile.*

The reproductive organs are not among the *vital* organs—in that their malfunction is not fatal—but they are paramount.

*Thomas Szasz describes masturbation as a primary sexual activity of humans. In the 19th century, it was a disease. In the 20th, it is the cure, he said. Woody Allen, on the other hand, wonders how having sex with 'someone you love' can be a sin.

Some tribal communities are known to have a pre-marriage ceremony at which the sexual endowments of the boy are thoroughly examined and certified. In others, the virginity of the girl is checked.* The very continuance of the species depends upon the man and woman being in fine fettle reproductively. It is little wonder that sterility or barrenness is considered to be the biggest of misfortunes. The fact that in many cases the inability of a man to impregnate his wife is the real problem is something many men refuse to consider. It is presumed that virility and success in bed is enough evidence of male capability in producing an offspring, which of course isn't true.

Some of the most challenging cases a doctor must treat will be about those parts of the body which society has decreed we hide from public gaze and which in turn has led to an urge to reveal. Style statements in apparel aim to show that which modesty commands should stay covered. It is a curious thing though, for there is really no secret about any part of the body. Molestation, child sexual abuse and rape are the result of resentment borne from a feeling of inferiority. The segregation of sexes at an early age, hypocritical societal norms that inhibit boy-girl friendships, stark social inequities, racial and communal enmity—all of these cause envy, frustration, anger and hatred for those others, and act as triggers for perversion. Forced sex is an act of oppression and control. It happens during wars and riots and is often instigated by those in power. Merely punishing the guilty does not solve the problem. Regular, repeated discussions with every section of society might direct us towards a remedy.

*The methods used in such examinations are beyond the scope of this book.

28

Mothers, Daughters, Wives

The sfl triangle is one-half feminine. The animate world is largely halved by a dividing line but several million others fall into the differently gendered community which needs all the goodwill and support that others can give. Why is sex and gender so important to the well-being of an individual? I list some stories: the usual; the unusual.

Thayamma was a short, pale woman with thin, baggy ears and dainty fingers that clutch a red handbag. She was neatly dressed, polite and nervous. Headache, she said: headache that has plagued her for twenty-one years and will not go away. She has tried everything, seen doctors in many neighbouring towns, made offerings to temples and even had a scan that cost three thousand rupees.

I asked if she had any other problems, like the lack of sleep? 'Sleep? I shut my eyes but that's it. No sleep for three nights now.' How about appetite? 'I can't bear the sight of food. Simply I eat to fill my stomach.' Any other aches and pains? 'The legs are sore, and this elbow and shoulder…a pulling sensation, like electric current.' Any symptom I mentioned, she had it.

A physical examination revealed nothing. As for the tests she had undergone, a mild anaemia was the only problem, for which she had been treated. When I told her this, her lips trembled and her eyes became wet. 'My mother is afraid it is something serious,' she said. 'If something happens to me, there is no one to look after her. A diabetic...'

Thayamma had never married. Her three sisters and two brothers, all younger to her, were well settled. 'Our father died when I was twenty,' she said. 'I had to leave college and work.' It was a struggle, but she managed, until the diabetes and arthritis began to trouble her mother and she became bedridden.

Were her siblings not able to offer any help in looking after their mother? They did not. 'They have families of their own.' Her face brightened momentarily. 'And mother prefers to stay with me, in her own home.' With a little probing I found that her anxiety was about her own future after her mother's demise. The house would go to the older of her two brothers and as yet there had been no talk of how she would cope.

The family system that we are justly proud of has failed many a daughter such as this. Daughters who deny themselves their own dreams and devote themselves to utterly selfish parents may end up lonely, frustrated and often uncared for in their later years. Thayamma's persistent headaches are signals from her body, silent shrieks of protest against the implacable stresses of sacrificing everything for her mother's comfort. Women come to the clinic with vague symptoms like burning in the head, ringing in the ears, leg cramps, indigestion, nausea, giddiness, fainting spells. Ask leading questions, like 'Do you also see light flashing in one eye?' or 'Do your knees click?' and it is a 'Yes!' They are dying to be told that there is something seriously wrong with them—an instinctive longing to get some form of attention.

Men are not exempt from such unusual causes of stress. A not-so-young man appeared in my clinic complaining of neck pain. 'Nothing you give will help,' he said, boastfully. 'I've seen the best.' Since he had absolved me of any responsibility, we talked. And out it came. At forty-two, he was still in search of a wife. 'We have a farm, a comfortable house, a car. Enough in the bank, and a good social life. My mother has been looking and asking. Every girl wants to marry someone who will move to a city. But mother needs me, I cannot leave this place.'

I don't recall trying to treat his aching neck. But I did suggest that he find the girl himself, rather than wait for his mother to find one. Months later he came with an invitation to his wedding. When I met him recently, he thanked me, not for his matrimonial good fortune, but for helping him with the neck pain. 'I did not treat you,' I said, remembering.

'I know. But you told me to find a girl for myself and it wasn't all that difficult once I started trying. I no longer spend my evenings on an easy chair, watching television.'

Fashioned out of historically long periods of patriarchy, a woman's survival instincts are often secretive; or tragically slavish. Most of us leave home when we marry to live in another home, in another village, or town. We acquire a new name, a new set of family, by virtue of marriage. The husband, too, has new relatives but he does not change his name, or leave his home and live with the 'in-laws'. The compulsory dislocation of the newly married woman has begun to change, but the vast majority of us have accepted this drastic and permanent resettlement without a murmur.

Daughter-in-law (and mother, father, son, sister, brother similarly rendered by matrimony) is a term I detest. You become a daughter by law. Law does not enter the confines of a home. The change of circumstance begins the moment she steps over the threshold into her husband's home; she is pressed and compressed into place. Such containment is perceived to be for the good of the family and is not always insensitive or cruel. I remember the way my mother would always stand when her mother-in-law (our grandmother) entered the room. She would remain standing, even when they talked at length. As teenagers we balked at this custom. Mother did not change her ways, and our grandmother did not ask her to sit.

Here's an example which could be part of a survival kit for women in certain situations: Gayatri called one day, asking for an appointment. She was holidaying in our area and needed to see a doctor. A well-groomed, serious-looking woman entered my clinic at the appointed time. She started by saying, 'I'm a day's journey away from home. It's reasonably certain that I will not see you again and that's the reason I'm consulting you.'

She was the managing director of a medium-sized garment retail firm in Hyderabad and married for fifteen years to Dinesh, who was in the Indian Administrative Service. They had a three-bedroom independent house in Jubilee Hills where they lived with their two children and Dinesh's parents. Here was a modern Indian family which managed to get everything right. A good marriage, bright children, contented grandparents and economic prosperity. Even if you zoomed in, you would see no cracks. The pivot of this exceptional family is Gayatri. She supervises the domestic help and the gardener, does the weekly shopping, pays bills, helps the kids with their homework, takes her in-laws to the doctors' and attends functions with or without Dinesh. Dinesh is perfectly happy with the woman he married. His parents never fail to shower her with praise that is genuine. The kids, of course, love their mom.

'This is the life I wanted. I enjoy my job, my success, my family. The kids are at a summer camp, you know, it's a fabulous thing…' She lowered her gaze. 'The years go by, the demands keep increasing. They really never end, do they? Both my in-laws are now hard of hearing and I speak to their siblings and other relatives on their behalf. Which means I must note down significant events like birthdays and festivals, call them up (with father- or mother-in-law seated next to me) and speak for them, listen for them. It is exhausting and—and I don't like doing it.

'Holidays are the worst, there's so much that needs to be done. Take in-laws for blood tests, to the doctor's clinic or to the other end of the city to visit some relative, the children to the movies. "Please drop us there, Mom, and pick us up in two hours, okay?" Or Dinesh wheedling me with, "That neck-and-shoulder massage you gave me last time, it was simply the best…how about it?" I'm not blaming anyone but the more I do, the more they want. Dinesh makes much of the tensions at work and once home, he spends time with the kids, and his parents. He has plenty of time to relax. I am exhausted too, after a long day at the office and the hour's ride back home. But there are all those everyday needs of the family to fulfil. It has become so mechanical, I hardly have time to pause.'

'You could talk it over with your husband. Or his mother.'

'That's the most frustrating part. Dinesh listens, that's it. His mother gives me a hurt look. She tells me about her young days when she had to manage without the mixie or microwave, without convenience goods available in shops. The fact that I hold a full-time job with responsibilities is ignored.'

Gayatri paused, and looked defiantly at me. 'I began a silent, secret rebellion. I started doing things that gave me pleasure. After work on Saturdays, I would take a short detour to meet a friend for coffee and gossip. Or I would stop by in town to dawdle for a while, sit at some restaurant and watch people. If Dinesh or anyone else in the family called, I could always say, truthfully, that I was on my way home. I started to put away portions of my favourite food and ate it when no one was around. It wasn't easy. I ate when the family had gone to bed or sometimes feeling really greedy would eat in the bathroom.'

'Did that make you feel better?'

She shook her head. 'They are guilty pleasures. This year Diwali came with a weekend and it was four days off but I had to go on urgent work to Bombay. It was to do with some foreign business that the company could not afford to miss. Disappointment all round. Sympathy for me. I was elated. I flew not to Bombay (I had made up the story about a business trip) on any official trip but to Madras. I spent four glorious days doing my thing. A decadent afternoon in a beauty parlour, looking up friends, watching movies. Pampering myself! Sleeping!

'This, being here, is one such holiday. I feel dreadful at times, knowing I have become selfish, I'm scheming all the time. But I still do everything that my family needs.'

I observed her more closely, this woman who had revealed so much of her inner self to me. As she talked, her expression softened. A tender look came into her eyes. 'You must wonder why I came to you. I want to know what you feel about me, now that I have told you all this. Is it all very hateful? Please. I want to know.'

Fault her? For what? It did not seem likely that her husband or in-laws would sympathize with her if she told them what she had done. They would be hurt and probably very angry to hear that as wife and daughter-in-law she did not find contentment in fulfilling her duty and receiving appreciation from them. I told her, as cautiously as I could, that it was better not to tell her family. But it was necessary to make them understand her needs in an honest manner. To say: 'I need rest', 'I need to be by myself a bit', 'I feel the strain of taking on all these responsibilities.' There would be some friction and unpleasantness, perhaps, but it would be better to make them understand.

It is over a year or more now, and I have tried to understand Gayatri's situation by talking about it to some of my male friends. Their reactions were quite extraordinary.

'Children need their mother,' said one with the air of someone discovering a truth.

'Working women are too self-centred,' said another, as if he were not talking to one.

A third said that a woman should never forego the gentle, soft side of her nature which made her so special. 'This woman should be grateful to her husband and in-laws who allow her to go out and work,' he added.

One of my friends who has a working wife, stayed silent. I could almost read his thoughts: Could my wife be doing something like this? Six out of the seven men I talked to felt that Gayatri's actions were deplorable.

*

Couples anxious to have children visit infertility clinics. In many centres, they are either not told about the high rate of disappointment; or if they are told, they choose to ignore this possibility resulting in emotional and physical stress, besides the huge financial wallop of each try. Failure to conceive after elaborate treatment leads to dejection and marital disharmony. Society is much to blame for the perception that natural childbearing is essential to happiness. Adoption is a sensible and socially responsible action. A young couple telling their daughter she was adopted explained that it made her special compared to other kids, just as Sita was adopted by Janaka and Krishna was adopted by Yashoda. Thrilled, the girl ran off to tell everyone: 'I'm 'dopted!'

The whole drama of reproductive maturity starts early, when a girl begins to menstruate. She needs reassurance, and advice about hygiene to prevent any physical and emotional discomfort, besides infections. Social taboos and poverty come in the way of a normal adolescence. My older sister, the tomboy of the family, was excellent in every field of sports and athletics; I could not understand why she suddenly stopped joining the rest of us at play after school. A few years later it happened to me and I hated the whole process of coping with it.

The monthly 'period' is the regular shedding and regrowth of the inner layer of the womb, controlled by the female sex hormones. To presume that a young woman is unclean because of this very natural process is as absurd as rebuking a boy for the emission of body fluids, or the ejaculation of semen. Until recently (and even now in conservative households), the menstruating girl or woman had to live in a separate part of the house and not touch the utensils or anything in the kitchen. She could not participate in religious rituals or go to a temple. In our own family that was our only taboo. Inclined to wickedness, I disobeyed the rule when I turned sixteen. Standing before the deity Igguthappa Swamy in the temple, I was overcome with guilt and fear. No god struck me down or showed any wrath, so I realized that my instinct had served me well. Women go to doctors asking for tablets to postpone their periods, so that they could attend religious ceremonies. This chemical interference has after-effects on health, like future infertility and worse. I always advise women against such self-degradation with the taking of tablets to delay the normal biological process of menstruation. A few go away convinced; others seek out doctors who will oblige.

When I was a young girl, only a small percentage of women could afford sanitary napkins or pads. There is more awareness now, and many more Indian women use sanitary pads. The others make do with cloth that is used over and over again for months, maybe years. The use of cloth is fine as long as it is washed thoroughly and dried in the sun and replaced every few months. The biggest problem with its use is that women struggle to find some private corner of their homes where they can hang the washed piece of cloth to dry. Moisture in the cloth promotes fungal and other infections which spread into the reproductive tract, blocking the fallopian tubes which conduct the ovum or egg into the womb for fertilization. This is a common cause of reduced fertility. In recent years, the menstrual cup has gained popularity and it might be a better alternative to pads. However, until we have entirely biodegradable, safe and affordable means of protection during periods, the disposal of used items is a huge problem.

It is imperative for civilized communities to shed these customs which are clearly hurtful to the physical and emotional well-being of women. Hindu women whose intellect is blunted by religiosity are indignant when their bolder sisters defy oppressive customs. Every religion sheds congealed traditions and moves forward alongside civilization. A lot of muck has flowed beneath the bridge since this comedy of errors began to play at Sabarimala (a hill named after a woman!). If women of a certain age are to be barred from entry to this temple, then men of a certain age must also be barred. They produce body fluids too, so how are they any cleaner or purer?

*

About the conditioning of gender bias, an incident from years ago comes to mind. My sister, who is married to an army officer, delivered a child in the early hours of the morning. Elated that all had gone well, my father sent a telegram to her husband, then a young captain on a posting in Kota, Rajasthan. 'V—— delivered a baby boy early this morning at 4.25 a.m.'

The telegram was collected by the captain's baat man—the flunkey who ensures that army officers are always comfortable and well turned out. He went about with downcast eyes and a gloomy face for a while before handing over the telegram to the father. 'Saab, I'm so sorry it is a baby and not a baba.'

That was more than four decades ago and the baat man might be excused for his gender bias. But the hankering for a male child is still prevalent among Indians, never mind their educational levels or economic status in society. Recently a young journalist found out that her parents had tried to abort her, because she was the second child and they wanted a boy. She had found out accidentally, when her mother asked her to sort out her old letters and preserve one from each friend or relative. The girl had chanced upon a letter written by her aunt, advising her mother to go to the town they lived in to have the abortion. The words were, 'Do it soon, or you will end up with another girl to marry off, and no one to look after the family business.'

I listened to the girl in absolute quiet. Those many years ago, her parents had come to me for a termination of the pregnancy, having found out the sex of their second child. They did not like what I told them, and remained cold towards me ever since. Their daughter, who almost did not happen, is bright and ambitious. She will be all right in spite of her unfortunate parenthood.

29

From 11 November 2016…

'Think as yourself, Dum-dum. Be yourself. That's all there is to life.'—VN

I put off writing this chapter, knowing it has to be written. The why of it will be clear to me when I have finished.

There have been moments in my life when I was saved from falling off the too-thin branch of a tree I should not have climbed. I was helped back to safe ground—by father, mother, husband, friend, teacher, stranger. All these years as I have talked to people, or conversed with my younger self, I have not stopped asking the same question: *how to live? One person helped me more than any other in coming close to finding an answer.*

Partnership in love is a process of discovery. I was attracted to Vijay by his ability to always stay in touch with his true self, to never say anything he did not mean. This cleanness of mind was natural to him. We met, we married and we lived together for twenty-three years. He was younger, wiser; gifted. He was my muse even before I met him; even before I heard about him.

Vijay never, ever behaved like he was special. Mrs Manson, the English teacher he revered at school, told me that he was miles ahead of any other student she had taught. All along, he read avidly, gorging on books by day, and often by night, with a torch beneath the coverlet, or in the toilet. His high-school years were not particularly happy. Knowing what it is to live within the framework of society and frustrated by its phoniness, he struggled to fulfil his obligations. With great reluctance, he gave in to his parents' choice of engineering as the most suitable profession for their only son. His passion was for the social sciences: there was no one to help him argue his case and he did not know how to rebel. 'We lived a sheltered, predictable, middle-class life,' he said. 'I was used to doing my duty. It made me too passive.' He would tell me this over and over again and mostly, without bitterness.

Vijay did have an excellent upbringing. His parents loved reading and scholarship. Fully aware of his exceptional merit, they encouraged him to read widely, to do well in school and to engage in every activity offered to students. When I first met his family, I was surprised by the lack of gendered inequality. Vijay and his father regularly helped clear the table after a meal, washed the dishes, cut vegetables and ironed clothes. They also respected tradition and followed its edicts.

So this 'only son' opted for mechanical engineering at the Indian Institute of Technology in Madras. The teaching was top-notch. Vijay was an eager participant in all activities like quiz contests, cricket, football and table tennis. He was a member of the editorial board of a college newsmagazine. I have with me several copies of the magazine, sent by one of the co-editors. 'Vijay wrote the editorial piece every time but insisted on putting the names of the rest of the team in the by-line,' he told me. Reading those typed sheets of *Focus*, I marvel at the boldness of its content. The quality of writing, though naive and rhetorical, is logical and impassioned. Vijay forged a deep friendship with a small circle of fellow-students, eight or ten of them, all brilliant and marvellously crazy in different ways. They met off and on, but remained close. For Vijay, these friendships were vital.

He had a lifelong fascination for the sciences and mathematics, but what truly delighted him were the social sciences. Literature was a passion. For a while he tried to fulfil expectations, to make something of what his parents had envisioned for him. However, it took no more than a few months in that hallowed institution for Vijay to accept that his being there was a terrible mistake: the eighteen-year-old apple of parental eyes began his life-long battle with depression. With it, came a journey of self-discovery. He immersed himself in books, stubbornly refused to attend classes and just about scraped through the first few years. In the fourth year, he dropped out of college, with the dean endorsing his decision, to the utter dismay of his family.

The year that followed was tough. He coped with his own sense of dejection, and the censure of his family. He contemplated suicide. A year went by: a girl he had met in college came back into his life. Thanks to her efforts, he landed work as a writer with an independent magazine, *The City Scan* in Delhi, founded by Probir and Aruna Dasgupta. Probir, as lovable as he is irascible, set high standards for his publication. The eager young apprentice learnt from him everything there was to know about journalistic work: writing, editing, printing and publishing; the absolute need for integrity and quality in reportage. Ananda Swaroop, who was one of a handful of youngsters who worked with Vijay, relates how he was assigned his first piece of work. He had been given a deadline which he missed; and continued to miss week after week. A furious Probir hauled him up and explained, in lush language, how he would react if the work wasn't completed in forty-eight hours, adding that he would be fired. Next morning, a neat typescript lay on the table before him. 'It was a fantastic piece,' says Probir. 'I remember saying, "We *have* to keep this guy!"'

Working for *City Scan* was sheer good fortune. Vijay learned fast. His work rarely needed editing; it covered literature, politics, travel, art, and journalism itself. It was the best of times; it was also the worst of times, for he took to drinking. The malady which befriended Vijay in his mid-twenties, remained with him for the rest of his life, leading to broken relationships, family tensions and driving mishaps. When we met, Vijay was already known for his eloquent poetry, as for his love of the bottle. All along he remained close to his family; at least close enough. 'They do not understand me,' he would say. 'But I don't blame them…' He was a dutiful son—more or less—but his real duty was to himself, of that he was certain. His family always came to his aid when he needed them, which was often enough.

Vijay's brilliance and his fascinating mindscape were also his disability. He bore his gifts, like his burdens, quietly. Those close to him know that he suffered from an utter lack of phoniness. He never grudged others their choice in life, as long as they did not mess with his. His only despair was against the world he lived in. The family—his parents and two sisters—bore the brunt of that despair.

Nearly a quarter of a century was witness to our marriage, our love. If this partnership is an equation, then I am that mirrored half which was awakened, thrilled, outraged, saddened, melted and moulded by the presence of one tormented by his gifts, and the despair that came with it. A deep awareness—of the worth and the worthlessness of life—crowned his gifts. It was a heavy crown and the only way he could lighten its weight was with the forgetfulness induced by drink. For those brief periods, he said, he was light and free.

I am a clever person myself, but not gifted; I'm purposeful and defiant, struggling to reach where I want to go. My quest has always been *How am I to do such-and-such?* Vijay's, *Why should I?* We had raging fights from which we emerged, feeling foolish, because often neither of us could recollect what had set it off. We talked, and how. About prose and poetry, politics, communities, religion, doctoring, kids, sex, love, films and all else that defines living. He never failed to stimulate me with his knowing and his simple goodness.

He would listen quietly to my implorations: *Write more. Publish more.* If success was not important to him, his writing was important to those who read him. 'It should be your mission in life, you nut-head, you idiot from somewhere, you-you…'

We can bypass the decorative words. I begged; I pleaded; I sulked; I threatened; I fought. Vijay went on doing what he did, and remained his ever-charming, stubborn, cussed, wise, foolish, beautiful self.

*

'I have a pain in my throat,' he said one day. Coming from a person who uses his words with faultless precision, I should have been warned. He did not say, 'I think I'm getting a sore-throat.' He said, 'I have a pain in my throat.'

'Since when?'

'I've been feeling it for some time,' and then he misled me with, 'It's probably nothing. Give me some tablets. It'll go.'

I flashed a torch into his throat. It looked fine. There were no associated symptoms like a stuffy nose, headache, fever or cough.

'Let's hope it's nothing serious,' I muttered.

'You mean—'

'In a smoker-drinker, yeah. Cancer is a possibility, I've told you a hundred times. More common is peptic oesophagitis. We'll see.'

Vijay bragged about his enviably good health, declaring that the poisons in his body kept the germs away. He loved his drink and his cigarettes a bit much. He did not smoke inside the house, but walked out to the balcony or the garden. He smelled each cigarette before lighting and preserved every used matchstick which we used to light the twin stove top. I still have three or four boxes of his used matches. We have known hard times, and it made us careful about money, often in foolish ways. Vijay kept a record of the number of cigarettes smoked each day and the average for the week, the month, the year. It ranged from 6.5 to 12.8 cigarettes a day, having decreased from his initial 18 plus. He was particular about the timing of every cigarette: soon after morning coffee, post-breakfast, after tea, before lunch… I never could keep track of these rigid norms and it would rile him now and then.

Drinking had its own system. He decided the day and time, (*usually*), after talking it over with me. Sometimes I protested, too feebly I think, knowing that his mind was made up and it meant a needless argument that would end in his favour. So if he said, 'I want to drink on Tuesday,' I'd say, 'Um. How much?' In our early years of marriage I protested, and preached about the hazards to health. 'I know,' he would say, most agreeably. His view was that it was his body and he was doing it with full awareness of the dangers. There was no point worrying about it.

The pain in his throat came and went at first and then it settled to a minor whinge. On 11 November 2016, we drove to Mysore and met Dr Harindra, an Ear, Nose and Throat (ENT) surgeon and colleague. It was late afternoon when Vijay drove our bright red Maruti Swift through the gates of Apollo Hospital; parking was easier than usual. We were talking about how we would spend the evening after the consultation. Minutes later, we met the doctor. He looked into Vijay's throat with an endoscope and nodded grimly at me. Vijay did not miss the glance.

'Tell me everything,' he said. He asked about treatment options. Half an hour later, we were on our way back to Hotel Govardhan where we stay when visiting Mysore. We did not speak.

In the room, Vijay said, 'Let's go down and get some coffee.'

We followed our usual routine: watched some television, read the papers, solved a quiz. Even at home, evenings were the best part of any day. For Vijay more so with a drink in hand.

'I'm not afraid, Kavu,' he said. 'Believe me. I'm not afraid of cancer, or of death. I don't want to suffer too much, though.'

Thinking we could leave for Bangalore the next day, I fixed an appointment at Apollo Cancer Hospital. Vijay demurred. He wanted a few days back at home 'to prepare himself'. A week later the biopsy and other tests were done to confirm the disease and its extent. It was still in the early stages and radiation treatment for seven weeks was the best option. The doctor was confident that there was an 80 per cent chance of a cure.

There are situations in life we do not expect, like a son telling his aged parents, 'I have cancer.' Vijay's family had moved to Bangalore when his father retired and lived there since. I remember that chill November evening, the sombre countenance of his father as he received the news, and the utter bleakness of 'What now?' from his mother who, along with his sisters, had been planning a celebration-lunch for Vijay's birthday which was the next day.

This was the momentous time when our prime minister announced an unforgettable gift: the banning of high currency notes and the promise of wiping out black money. I had a difficult week, with long hours in a queue at the bank, until Vijay's family bailed us out. We rented a room close to the hospital, on a squeezed-up alley, with just enough road amidst a mish-mash of urban living. We stayed there for seven weeks, cooking with a small stove placed on a table next to a television which offered some diversion. Vijay's treatment started a day after his birthday and comprised radiation treatment every morning and chemotherapy once a week. A middle-aged man from Bangladesh, undergoing the same treatment as Vijay had rented a room next to ours. At half-past seven every morning,

I would knock on his door and he would come along with us to the hospital, with Vijay driving. His young nephew who had accompanied him from Bangladesh, came too. As he was a college student, his time was the most expendable. He appeared to be more worldly-wise than his uncle and did most of the talking. They were farmers from a village near Dhaka and had sold a portion of their paddy fields in order to afford the treatment. The hospital had been recommended by a relative. They were satisfied with what they got, but often we saw them studying some bill, with deep concern and puzzlement.

Vijay walked into the hospital with cheerful acceptance. Being naturally friendly, he got on well with the staff, particularly the nurses. He joked in Malayalam, talked about movies, and there was an instant melt. We looked forward to the weekly visit his parents' home, to good food and the quiet comforts which only family can provide.

Seeing my husband suffer the effects of cancer and the consequences of treatment was a new experience for me. Until a few decades ago, general surgeons had the skill and the experience to tackle many cancers: breast, prostate, kidney, stomach, colon, thyroid, skin, bone, uterus, ovary, testes and the penis were a part of general surgical territory. In hospitals beyond the cities, it stayed so until recently. Excision of the tumour was the mainstay of cancer treatment, with radiation and chemotherapy being used as adjuncts. Knowing is not always an advantage. I stayed with Vijay through every day of his illness but I also ghost-walked with the medical team as they trooped together during ward-rounds; I listened in on their conversations, peered through glass-paned partitions at the strange scene of Vijay lying within the radiation chamber, his head encased in a plaster cast that had been moulded over his face, the powerful rays angled at the cancer cells. During the course of chemotherapy, I cheered silently as the chemical agents dripped into his veins and raced towards the targeted cells which would grimace and die. Good, good, good. At night I listened to his breathing and tried to quell my fears.

Care is taken during radiotherapy to safeguard normal cells, but some amount of damage to the neighbouring tissues is inevitable. Vijay was fifteen days into treatment when my sister and her husband came to see him. He was happy to see them and talked to them without discomfort but that was the last time he spoke without difficulty. Soon after, swallowing became painful and his taste buds began to wear out. His voice grew hoarse and he began to cough at night; saliva, which is essential for speech and swallowing, became dry and sticky, it clung to the back of the throat in strands and aggravated the cough. He gargled five times a day with bicarbonate of soda. In spite of medications and sitting propped up on pillows at night, he could not sleep. He became downcast and grumpy.

We read, played word-games and scribbled notes along the edges of newspapers or in a notebook which we used to record our daily expenses. Crossword puzzles (the tougher the better) were his favourite. I was not accustomed to Vijay being sick. It was he who nursed me back from any sickness, made tea, massaged my back while relating 'the best' of rugby jokes or reciting poems. By the end of the third week, he could taste nothing. He lost his voice completely. The margins of newspapers filled up:

'Throat is painful.'

'Difficult to sit up all night.'

'When do I get the next painkiller?'

'Left nostril hurting. Ask the doctor if I can get something stronger for pain. I took the tablet at 6.10…'

'Why aren't you listening to me…? I know you're tired, but you're not listening to me.'

'Stop telling me to eat.'

Being witness to his suffering were the worst moments of my life. I saw his body shrink; I saw him suffer. Two of his cousins had made arrangements to send soft and nourishing food to the hospital with the hope of stimulating his taste buds. It seemed to help for a while but soon I was eating most of it.

When the seven weeks of radiation treatment was over, the doctor reassured Vijay. 'The taste will come back within a week, and you will begin to feel normal.' We were happy enough to buy several boxes of the best quality sweets for all the medical staff who were involved in his treatment.

Vijay couldn't wait to be home. He loved long-distance driving—stopping on the way for dosa, competing with me in antakshari, which invariably ended in hostilities. This time, he readily agreed that we should hire a driver.

Once home, we regained our connections with everyday life. Having stayed away for two months I felt keenly the loss of the essential link I have with patients, and was happy to get back to work. In the evenings we sat on the balcony upstairs and looked at the untended garden in furious bloom. We talked (me mostly) or we read; we absorbed the silence. I waited for the day when he would eat properly. With smoking and drinking denied, it was hard on him. At times he sneaked in a cigarette and was immediately repentant. 'Don't leave any cash lying around,' he told me. Two weeks went by. He began to speak in a hoarse whisper but the taste buds struck work for two-and-a-half months; the pain worsened. 'I dread the thought of eating,' he said. 'Don't force me.' He grew irritable. The radiotherapist suggested stronger painkillers, a sedative and cough suppressants; he said it was a matter of time. We decided that perhaps he could stay with his parents for a while. His mother's cooking being infinitely superior to mine would surely help. So Vijay went to Bangalore while I stayed back.

A week later he sent me a message. 'Can't manage. I think I want out…I need you here.'

I went. The journey seemed to take forever. Vijay greeted me at the gate. He was smiling. The shock of seeing him after a long week, and observing the cruelty with which the disease was consuming him, cut deep; cut sharp. The following day he was seen by the ENT surgeon at St John's Medical College Hospital and admitted for a detailed evaluation. There was severe infection in the irradiated area which had unfurled sideways, causing swelling around the windpipe, the gullet and the voice box. The need for a tracheostomy—an opening made into the windpipe to safeguard his breathing—was absolute and urgent.

The hospital is attached to the medical college campus where I studied, where I participated in seminars, lectures and readings; and where in the Department of Humanities, Vijay and I had given creative-writing lessons to students. That day, the short journey, as I walked beside the stretcher along sanitized passageways, the swing doors and lifts to the operating theatre is one of the gravest I have endured. I was very nervous. Vijay's sister came and for an hour-and-a-half, we sat outside the theatre complex. When it was over the surgeon explained that the infected material around the cancer site was extensive and ominous of advancing disease. The biopsy, however, proved negative. Still, he cautioned me that this often happened when the cells were too damaged for the typical features of cancer to be seen. A pathologist friend in the US whose opinion I trust told me that the chances of cure were not as good as originally predicted.

With the infected material cleared away, Vijay felt better. The pain lessened, the cough disappeared and he could speak a few hoarse words, by closing the tracheostomy opening. Since he could not be fed anything by mouth until the swelling inside subsided, a feeding tube had been inserted through the nose and past the throat into his stomach. Clear liquids were fed through this naso-gastric tube, thus keeping the afflicted area free. The swelling inside the throat persisted even after a week, and it seemed likely that the tracheostomy would have to stay for weeks or months. The feeding tube that passed through his nose could be replaced by one placed directly in the stomach or in the small bowel for greater comfort and better nutrition with a wider tube.

I met the surgeon who was to do this procedure. He scheduled it for the following day and added that he was the best surgeon in the hospital and so Vijay was in safe hands. I remember feeling puzzled by this statement. A feeding jejunostomy is a simple surgery, simpler than a tracheostomy. It took no longer than twenty or thirty minutes. Vijay was fully conscious and smiling as he was wheeled out.

'The anaesthetist is Dr Mary's daughter,' he said to me. 'Her name is Anjali.' Mary is a friend from my college days who later served as the dean of our medical college.

When Vijay was given water through the intestinal tube next day there was distension and discomfort, indicating that the normal peristaltic action which squeezes food through the digestive canal had not returned. Surgical interventions in the abdomen, big or small, will cause a temporary shutdown of the normal peristaltic activity, usually for twelve to twenty-four hours; at times, longer.

The twenty-four hours stretched to two, three, four days. The distension persisted. The intestines were silent, inactive, off-duty. Nine anxious days passed and still the low rumble of normal gut that doctors listen to with the stethoscope was absent. I was distraught and fearful, in spite of constant reassurance from the team of doctors who came at least once a day, listened with their stethoscopes and went away. The intravenous fluids were unable to provide the required calories or nutrition. Vijay was being starved.

On the ninth day he had a dark-brown, 'coffee-ground vomitus' which portends major distress within the bowel; in his case, a possible blockage. It was operating-day for the surgeon and his entire unit was busy inside the theatre. The nurses said they could do nothing beyond conveying a message to the surgeon over the phone, and no, none of the doctors from another surgical unit, or I, could suggest any treatment. I was upset and angry. At four in the evening, eight hours after Vijay started to vomit, I went to the theatre complex myself, and insisted that Vijay be seen immediately. It is the only time I have done such a thing, and hopefully the last.

Dealing with the relatives of patients can be difficult. They might ask irrelevant questions, insist on the guarantee of a complete cure, address you as a god, or become downright offensive and threatening. The most frustrating are those who do not listen, or try to understand what is being explained. They come back day after day with the same questions. It can get to you, particularly at the end of a tiring day of work. I have learnt not to interfere in the work of other medical professionals. Having reposed trust in a doctor, I keep my surgical self within me and listen to the one in charge. It is not mere courtesy, but a clearing of space. The doctor should not feel pried upon. It works well (most of the time). But this ordeal was like no other.

Half an hour later the surgeon came, along with the rest of his team. I related the events of the day. 'We will refer him to the gastroenterologist,' he said, gruffly.

'Surely, the vomiting is related to the surgery?' My voice might have risen a few decibels. 'He's been vomiting since morning and you did nothing. Now you want him to wait for another doctor?'

'Madam, he's not my only patient. 'I have been very busy all day. In fact, I have just operated on a VIP—'

'This happens to be *my* VIP!'

'If you're unhappy with the treatment, I can refer your husband to another surgeon.'

'*You* operated on him. It is *your* responsibility to handle any complication.'

He did not like the way I spoke. The assistant surgeons and postgraduate trainees and interns were all there, along with the nurses. He muttered instructions to his team and left. The next day a CT scan of the abdomen showed a total blockage of the intestine, most probably due to an adhesion. Usually, adhesions cause a partial block and can be treated without surgery, but this was total. He would have to undergo surgery yet again, to unblock the gut. Vijay would be taken to the OT for the third time in three weeks. It hurt me to think that this had nothing to do with his primary illness, it was a complication of the previous surgery, a simple one, of inserting a tube into his bowel. Such things happen. It isn't anybody's fault. But to shrink from one's responsibilities at such a crucial moment, is.

I explained the problem to Vijay, and he did not demur. I stayed (outwardly) calm. It was late evening on the 9th of June 2017. He was lying on the operating room stretcher in the waiting area of the theatre complex. I could feel the contours of his facial bones as I stroked his face. He gripped my hand in his, the hand I reach out for every time, now thin and wasted. He stroked my face. 'I love you,' he said, a smile shining in his eyes.

His mother and sister were away in Kerala. Three of his cousins were prompt with help, the immediate cash payment as required was made. We waited outside the entrance to the operating theatre. Three hours later—it was half-past ten in the night—I was beckoned to the waiting area. The surgeon came, visibly tired, his voice subdued. 'The abdomen was riddled with adhesions. I cannot figure out why. It was such a clean abdomen when we did the feeding-jejunostomy.' I took in the meaning of his words. It had been a difficult surgery. He had spent hours patiently freeing the delicate loops of bowel from the web-like adhesions that made the loops stick together in an impossible maze and blocked the lumen of the gut. 'Now we must wait and hope,' he added, gravely. 'Please pray that all goes well.'

I wiped my cold, sweating face and went to tell the others.

Next day: Vijay seated in a chair by the bed in the post-op ward, in pale blue pyjama-shirt, looking very pleased. 'Did it go well? I don't feel so bad.' The first day after a major surgery patients tend to be cheerful because the pain-relieving effects of anaesthesia and strong medications are still at work. Then followed another long wait for the peristalsis to return. The effects of prolonged under-nourishment in a person afflicted with a serious illness are grim. Vijay was exhausted; he lay in bed, listless, without the strength to read. *Not to read.* Vijay was at least a-book-a-day person, now he could not even finish a page.

A few more days, the doctors said. We must wait. His temperature spiked every day and was frequently heralded by rigors. 'I can feel the shivers coming. Stroke me…' he would whisper and curl his weak body inside several blankets. I held him down and reached for the call-bell. Doctors are not around always, they cannot be, they have plenty to do. When you need them, they are somewhere else. I was tired of pleading with nurses, entreating the ayah to bring a change of sheets, tired of checking the tubes, wound dressings, the urinary catheter, the fluid dripping into his veins. I went to the pharmacy twice or sometimes thrice a day to purchase intravenous fluids, antibiotics, painkillers, catheters, tubes, dressings, ointments, lotions, sometimes at night after ten when only the main pharmacy would be open and it was a long bleak trudge through the corridors to the ground floor. Relatives and friends came, all of them full of kindness and affection; they stayed; they went. Days and nights merged in a haze. Late in the night I lay in bed, my stomach full of swallowed tears. I was exhausted, hurting everywhere from sleeping on the narrow couch meant for the patient's attender and sleep was constantly interrupted—all of it routine for one who attends a sick person in hospital.

During those most distressing weeks, we found a friend in

the pain therapist, a doctor with the ability to connect with the patient. She spoke to Vijay as a person, and not just an illness to be treated or a problem to be solved. It is the most valuable asset a doctor can bring to the bedside of one who is suffering all over. I remember how we looked forward to her visits, and to those of the ENT specialist, who was always kind and gentle. He too was a very busy surgeon and his outpatient department teemed with patients every day, but he made it a point to attend to all patients with equal concern. And there were two doctor-friends from the community health department, who offered any assistance I might require.

One night, sometime between 1 and 2 a.m., Vijay became disoriented, got off the bed and walked out of the room, resulting in the many tubes that were attached to him getting ripped off. Blood and fluid everywhere, nurses in panic and Vijay standing in one corner of the room, like the bewildered victim of an ambush. The senior nurse was shouting at him, another called the doctor on duty, patients and attendants from adjacent rooms crowded at the door.

Vijay asked, in complete innocence: 'What happened, Kavu…? Someone pulled off all my tubes…'

We got him back in bed. The tubes were reconnected and the intravenous lines set up.

'A complete mystery,' Vijay murmured, as we wiped away blood stains and changed his clothing. 'You know the Jesuit priests, you should get them to investigate this case. They're clever, and good at solving such cases.'

I stayed up for what remained of the night, lying next to him, stroking his back. I realized what the problem was: he had not been given his routine anti-depressants for some time. He was on morphine tablets for pain and it had been decided that it would be enough while he was in hospital and still off oral feeds. It took two days to decide the best course of treatment. The pain-therapist and the psychiatrists had to concur regarding efficacy and safety in using multiple drugs. As soon as it was sorted out, Vijay began to stabilize, and slept soundly thereafter.

He continued to spike fever which was mostly likely due to sepsis. I requested that the senior physician see him. He was prompt in doing blood, urine and wound cultures, after which higher antibiotics were prescribed; and a central line inserted into a large vein near the collar bone to feed him with high-calorie fluids. Vijay had five tubes piercing his body which needed care at all times of day and night. Cleaning, suctioning and dressing the tracheostomy site, measuring and emptying the urine, change of dressings, positioning the three intravenous lines, the injections, blood transfusions, the innumerable daily pricks. Even with the high-calorie fluids, he could get no more than 800 calories a day.

Nine days after the third surgery, the bowels began to wake and the first faint tinkle of peristalsis was heard through the stethoscope. Fluids were dripped into the intestinal tube in small amounts and slowly increased. Within four or five days, Vijay could manage a litre-and-a-half of liquid diet. Such a relief. My own anger had subsided. The infection was controlled and Vijay felt better each day. But he was fearful of anyone of the general surgical team approaching him and would insist I stay by his side every time. Not once through all his trials was he difficult or disagreeable: for that trait, I reluctantly take the credit.

Vijay was on the mend and we were hopeful of being out of the hospital. For some days, when I made a short trip home by myself to settle some urgent matters. During that time his friends and family took over. One of his close friends stayed in the hospital at night and others filled in during the day. It is not easy to give this kind of sustained assistance, taking off from work or leaving behind other duties, travelling through the madly impossible traffic to be with someone who needs a lot of help. One evening, Vijay was wheeled into the garden and taken around the hospital campus. He would tell me about it many times, how good it was to feel the breeze, to look at everyday life. A writer friend came, hauling a heavy bag full of books. He spoke to Vijay for two hours about all that was happening in the writers' world; he implored Vijay to stay positive. A day or two before we were to leave for home, there was a call from Delhi: some of his colleagues from the *City Scan* days of three decades past were taking a flight into Bangalore to see him. Vijay had lost 25 kilos in weight and was very weak. But that day when they came, he walked to the hospital cafeteria where we sat drinking coffee, talking precious trivialities. He told them, 'I never cared too much about food but now I crave for a masala dosa.' There is a clear image in my mind of him seeing his friends off to the cab back to the airport, a wide grin taking over his thin face as he hugged them goodbye.

A few days with his family and then the long ride home. It was marvellous, in spite of the time-regulated chores—dressings, preparation of feeds (seven times a day), the medications. Vijay tuned in without fuss. We had also started a natural, seaweed-based supplement to boost his immunity. He began to gain weight, he walked, and two weeks later, began to drive short distances. He started to read again, and it rejuvenated him more than any food. It felt good to see him forever scanning the bookshelves, suggesting books for me to read. He drank small amounts of tea, coffee, water; ate a soft-boiled egg.

I was delighted.

'Custard? Khichdi? Porridge?'

He shook his head. 'I'll take it slowly.'

He sat on a chair in the bathroom, wearing my light mauve raincoat to keep away the chill, while I bathed him in sections. It exhausted him. Scrubbed, dried and clothed he would grip my hand. 'It's hard on you, Kavu.'

Golden weeks they were. Only I was just too occupied, with

all the exertions, the planning and thinking of what was to be done next. I did not dwell enough on the pleasure of seeing Vijay regain his wholeness except during brief moments when we sat together on the balcony upstairs. It is where he sat every day, reading; smoking; drinking; at peace. 'Come sit, come sit,' he would say to me in the evenings. One of his perpetual grouches was that I did not spend enough time with him, that I rushed about being busy. In trying to finish my endless chores before seizing the moments on the balcony, I ended up with too little time for the person I loved.

I was determined to see the back of his illness. He had suffered too much, but now he was confident, his face serene and untroubled, his smile weak but real. I got in touch with the chief of head and neck surgery at the Tata Memorial Hospital in Bombay, sent him the documents of Vijay's illness and sought his advice on the future course of management. Surgery to extirpate remnant cancer tissue is an option, he said, because it was quite likely that residual disease was present. Instead of going to Bombay in Vijay's weakened condition, he suggested we see a surgeon he could recommend in Bangalore. He phoned and got us an appointment. So we set out once more from home: I prepared myself for the possibility of surgery.

Vijay told me, clearly, that he would go through the required tests but would not have any more surgery. 'Keep an open mind,' I said.

Throughout the six-hour journey I was restless and brooding. I imagined the inside of his throat, the little cul-de-sac called the pyriform fossa where malevolent cells multiplied, in a frenzy of self-mutilation and destruction of the normal: advancing, assaulting, constricting. The neck is the vital highway that connects head—the abode of thought, memory, intellect, emotions and the senses, the summation of the person one is—with the rest of his body without which, one is not. The neck is also the conduit for air, food and the vital channels of blood which traverse the neck between the heart and the head. The packed but well-regulated highway had to make room for a mob on a rampage, invading and lynching without reason. The emperor of maladies, indeed: an emperor who needs the victim for his own survival.

I pulled myself back to what needed to be done. If surgery were advised, and if I could convince Vijay to have it, how extensive would the excision be, how easy or difficult to protect the vital structures? What if, what if…?

We were happy to stay this time with the warm and fun-loving family of Vijay's cousin. Vijay was relaxed, smiling. The following day we went to see the surgeon he had been referred to. The evaluation took two days: the tracheostomy was checked and the feeding tube in his intestines replaced with a fatter tube through which thicker fluids could be fed. During the course of the evaluation, a counsellor asked Vijay, 'Do you feel fear about your illness?'

'Fear, no; anxiety, yes,' was his emphatic answer. 'I'm anxious about surgery.'

When she probed further, he said he had decided that he would not be cut up again.

The tests came back negative for recurrence or spread. The disease was quiescent.

'Concentrate on improving your nutrition and strength,' the surgeon said. 'Come back for a review in three months.' We were overcome with relief; we rested awhile and drank tea at the cafeteria before leaving the hospital.

Six or seven of Vijay's friends from college days turned up that evening. Vijay reclined on a couch, quiet merriment lighting up his face as he listened to their banter, mostly about their capers in college. Late evening when they left, he walked to the lift to see them off. 'Now I'm tired…' he said, beaming nevertheless. Early next morning on 31st July, we returned home.

30

…to 9 August 2017

Happiness!

All day I hurried about, doing what needed doing. The bigger feeding tube helped tremendously; now I could feed him better food, more food. The progress was unmistakable—a spring in his step, some strength in the shoulders, a quickness of eye. The following week, on the 5th of August, was our wedding anniversary. A young student from Harvard was on a visit and had been with us all day. We dropped him at the town bus-stand in the evening and then went up to our balcony to celebrate. Vijay had a drink and a cigarette. There was no denying him that small pleasure. I babbled like I do when I'm excited. 'We'll go somewhere on a short-short holiday. Mangalore or Mysore?'

'Not so soon, Dum-dum… I want to be well enough for the dosas.'

That day he repeated what he had told me dozens of times: 'I'm not afraid of death, K. I'm worried about you.'

'Now who's the idiot?'

8 August 2017

We drove about 15 kilometres to buy a few things we needed, including organic manure which we buy by the sack for our garden. I asked a young man at the store to load it into the car.

Vijay, who had been waiting at the wheel, said: 'Can we go home now? I feel weak.' So I decided not to stop for the other purchases and we headed home, stopping on the way for a cold lemon drink for Vijay. He drank it down and immediately felt better.

'Go ahead, buy the other stuff. I'm okay.'

Back home, he lay down and rested for half an hour.

9 August 2017

I woke at 5 a.m. or so, make the fine gruel for Vijay. He was up by then. I cleaned his wounds, changed the dressing over the tracheostomy and the belly; I gave him the first of his tube feeds (by now reduced from eight to six larger feeds) and only then did he get to drink his coffee. That day as usual, a little before nine, he drove me to the clinic, stopping on the way for three girls on their way to school. Vijay loved to offer rides to old ladies, schoolteachers, labourers, the telephone linesman, the good-for-nothing layabouts, schoolkids, college students, the milkman, anyone. A few times the ride ended with a smiling beneficiary asking Vijay if he could please spare some cash?

It was an unusually busy clinic and I did not realize it was past one until Vijay appeared. Seeing that I hadn't finished, he said, 'Take your time, I'll wait.' That day he spoke to so many—the two barbers, the pharmacist, the ladies tailor, the bakery guy and some of the patients whom he knew. He told everyone he was better. I finished in less than an hour but was slightly irritable for some reason, maybe it was the fact that his feed had been delayed and there were some other things to be taken care of; maybe I was tired. Vijay was cheerful. He was teasing me about something and I barely listened. We rested awhile after lunch; I read the papers. It was half-past three when I finished giving him the fifth feed for the day. He was kidding about something, I was still edgy. At four, I went to the kitchen to make tea. 'Half a cup for me,' said Vijay coming up to me. 'Shall I switch on the computer?'

'Yeah, do that. I'll bring the tea.'

I heard him coughing in the toilet upstairs. It was not uncommon but when it persisted, I stroked his back. I went upstairs with the tea, placed the mugs on the computer table and went to the toilet. Vijay was bent over the sink, bringing up blood. It poured out of his mouth, nose and the tracheostomy site and around it. I held him tight, turned the tap on full, hoping to wash it away and noted with horror the *bright* unmistakable redness of arterial blood. Major haemorrhage.

'Viju, come lie down. We're going to the hospital…Viju!'

He shook his head weakly, but lurched the few steps to the bed. 'No don't lie down, sit up! Sit up!' I placed a bucket before him. I called my brother. 'Come now! I'm taking Vijay to Mysore. It's serious.' I was screaming. He understood. I heard him say, 'I'll come with you.' I was holding Vijay and trying to call a driver I knew, saying something in panic and as I spoke, Vijay fell away, his head striking the stool on which he had three books that he was reading. All Kipling. I lifted him onto the bed, let him recline, turned him to one side and realized he was not breathing. I tried; I tried. Vijay had tasted his last mouthful of air and closed his eyes.

I kicked the bed and fisted the wall and stamped my feet in my unspeakable and foolish sorrow. Maybe twenty minutes later I heard the car, went down the stairs. My brother and sister-in-law knew as soon as I opened the door, I think. They quietly took charge, got the doctor and started to make phone calls.

The house filled with people. What was I thinking, as I sat in our long front-room like a battered piece of furniture, words of solace swirling and drifting around me? I was overcome with the numbness shock and disbelief at the permanence of what had happened. I did as I was told. We would go to Bangalore the same night, reaching in the early hours of the morning. His mother, his sister, the extended family, friends, neighbours; the funeral. We subsided into a deep, collective grief. Permanently bereft, I was unable to keep pace with the process of mourning, although my physical self tried. On the third day I realized what I had to do. I explained to his family and started back for home.

To bleakness. To white walls and red flooring, the tiled roof which leaks in many places, our bedroom with its iron cot, the jumble-tumble, the spiders and the glow worms lost in the night, our magical balcony and the bats and owls that skim overhead on long winter evenings, the chaotic garden and the tulsi plant. The chillies, pumpkins, lilies and pineapple which he planted and left for me to tend, with him looking on from the balcony where he sat eternally. *Eternally.*

It is where I have to be.

*

This section of the book has been hard to write. While the rest of it is about doctors and my own career, this is about an exceptional life which could not be saved by the medical system. It is about the very personal, but the purpose of writing it is not personal.

The doctors did what they believed was best for Vijay. They extended care and cure within the limits of their own understanding and within the limits of a system which employs and empowers them. The end can be explained away as one of the outcomes of cancer which does, indeed, frequently kill, in spite of timely treatment. What I mean to do is go back to the first page of the story of Vijay's illness and see it again with the alertness it demands.

Vijay's illness was an education for me. I saw how doctors who work in big-sized institutions must sustain their concentration and quality of work all day, as they work through scores of patients. In living through the illness, I have, all along, been playing on both sides of the divide. The doctor-self was out there with the doctors, tagging along: listening, agreeing, doubting, debating, accepting or disputing. I was in the operating theatre, snooping while they dealt with the insides of my beloved: the snip-and-clamp, the suctioning of spilt blood, the sewing and the closure; I followed tubes as they invaded private passageways. Heavens, is this what the best of us surgeons do? Offer the doggedly pragmatic answer to everything by wielding the knife with acumen and varying degrees of artistry, taking away the offending stuff and putting together the remnants? I wrestle with my displeasure of our limitations. All the while we are also highly dependent on medicines which have been synthesized artificially and are known to help cure many an illness. In the end, it was only nine months of cancer. Did the powerful rays of radiation kill every one of the malignant cells in his throat and only those? Of course not. Some normal cells were also damaged or destroyed and replaced by fibrous scar tissue which is hard, unyielding and useless. I worried that this hardened mass, lying so close to the major blood vessels which traverse the neck to and from the head could be damaged. What then? I had asked the doctors about the risk of haemorrhage and was reassured that it was rare.

Rare, but not implausible?

'Put it out of your mind,' one doctor said.

The two hospitals where Vijay underwent the major portion of his treatment are the Apollo Cancer Hospital and St John's Hospital, both in Bangalore. It is unfair to both institutions to do a comparison. The Apollo Group is the pioneer of privatized, corporate health care. It has sustained its value for decades in a highly competitive medical industry. Corporate health care is a business venture, answerable to directors and shareholders; profit is the ultimate goal. The client pays for every expense—direct or indirect—incurred by the hospital in the process of treatment. Vijay's radiotherapy cost Rs 2.35 lakhs; the chemotherapy, laboratory and X-ray charges plus the medicines and our two-month stay took it to Rs 4.5 lakhs. We were satisfied with what we got.

Apollo Hospital and its cousins everywhere in the country are affordable to only about 15 per cent of us. They could reach more people by providing inexpensive basic medical services for ordinary ailments without the patient having to see a consultant and undergo innumerable tests; they could offer general-ward beds at cheaper rates, install inexpensive coffee- and tea-vending machines and provide affordable lodging services with simple provisions for cooking. A very large number of patients come from outside the city and will certainly look for such facilities so that a long-term stay for a patient does not also mean high living expenses for the attending relatives.

Corporate hospitals fall short in helping the average citizens, even when they undertake charitable services under Corporate Social Responsibility (the mandatory use of 2 per cent of profits on social welfare). The 2 per cent obviously pinches them hard—it is a lot of money. Determined to enhance self-image while appearing to do good, they resort to easy methods like conducting free medical camps and sending out mobile clinics and publicizing them with the use of banners, pamphlets, local newspapers and phone messages. The doctors deputed on such projects are not motivated for the work; it shows. Patients are checked in a cursory manner, prescribed token medicines and advised to go to their (city) hospital for tests and specialist consultations. In other words, it is a way of trapping more customers in the same net. For a medical camp to be successful, it is best to offer a definite service—like free cataract surgery, or simple day-case surgical procedures. If organized and conducted well, they are a great help.

A couple of decades senior to the Apollo group is St John's

Medical College and Hospital. It now covers the entire gamut of health care, with the 1800-bed hospital, medical college, nursing school, medical research, community health, outreach programmes and more. It is a hub of medical activity which works to full capacity, reaching out to the disparate classes that form our society. In my student days when Bangalore was smaller, this same space was well outside the city. Buses took no more than twenty minutes to take you to the city-centre. This area of Koramangala is now an entrepreneurial hub, with ceaseless traffic and construction work leading to unmanageable levels of noise and pollution.

The response from the public towards St John's has been warm and positive. I have used their facilities frequently, over the years. The doctors are committed, and work on fixed salaries, with fixed hours of private consultations permitted to senior consultants. The nurses are efficient, supremely confident and pleasant; the departments are well-equipped and adequately staffed. The community health programmes reach out to outlying villages and also help expose young trainee doctors to the problems of rural populations. The medical college is ranked among the best in the country.

I remain grateful to the ENT surgical team, the pain therapist and the physician for helping Vijay tide over this very difficult time of his illness. It was their caring as much as their efficiency which comforted him. Team-work is the hallmark of good service, and nowhere is it as crucial as in surgery. The biggest obstacle to a surgeon's success is the arrogance of believing that she or he has all the answers. And even if it is so, it should be revealed only through work. A surgeon must teach the juniors, trust them, and delegate duties. If a team works in fear and awe of the boss, they work only to impress and will never rise to their full potential. I am saddened to record this observation, and do so as an obligation to the institution which nurtured me in my years of training.

Vijay struggled all his life to fit into the normal order of living: he was a minority among minorities. His hospitalization and suffering filled me with bitterness and anger. The emptiness I wake up to each day is enriched only by my knowledge of him.

31

A Virus Strikes

The Covid-19 pandemic—which is ultimately connected to our careless handling of the environment—happened soon after I finished writing this book. Its publishing got delayed because of the virus and so it might be worthwhile to give it the importance it deserves.

When Covid-19 struck in March 2020, the Indian economy was already reeling from the tragic effects of demonetization. In addition, Kodagu had not recovered from being battered by floods and landslides for two consecutive years. Crops had been damaged, houses wrecked and tourism—a mainstay of Kodagu economy—was yet to recover fully. The lockdown in late March 2020 was imposed when we had just one positive case of Covid-19 in the district. So it was the lockdown that became our problem for several months. With no public transport, patients who suffered from chronic and acute ailments were unable to seek medical help. (On an average, our outlying villages are 5 to 15 kilometres away from any town which might have a chemist's shop, a public health centre, a nurse, or doctor.) Shop-owners, forced to shut down, took the brunt of the economic slide. A few shops remained open for about three hours a day but many essential provisions and medicines were in short supply. Vegetable vendors were temporarily shifted to an open maidan where they sat on the grass and sold less than fresh vegetables. Others, like those involved in road repairs or construction work, were left high and dry, as were school- and college-going students. Educating children through the digital medium proved to be an illusion in the villages, for only a small number of those with means could get some benefit from online classes.

In the early months of the pandemic, people were reluctant to take social distancing or the use of masks seriously. As for the hand sanitizer, everyone loved the idea of 'washing away' the virus with few drops of alcohol-scented liquid.* A cousin of mine along with her husband took the precautionary measures with complete seriousness and geared up before driving to the town to buy provisions: masked, gloved and goggled. They created a minor scene at the shops where everyone stared, unbelieving, at the pair of aliens.

The lifting of the lockdown in May 2020, which resulted in frenetic attempts to return to normal activity, caused a surge in Covid-19 cases. The following months saw their numbers increase to nearly 6000 cases in Kodagu. Patients were admitted to the district hospital in Madikeri, subjected to extensive tests, scans, isolation and treatment. Systematic surveillance and interaction with all the medical staff in the district were not done.

I shut the clinic, opened it, shut it again and finally decided to stay open. I lost about two months thus, but continued to see patients at home. Epidemiologists had warned that for each clinically confirmed case, there would be at least twenty more who were infected but asymptomatic. I tried to work within the confines of this crucial detail, did my own bit of clinical detective work in tracing persons who were most likely to be affected. I learnt about building immunity against the virus

*Soap works better, since its fatty content kills bacteria and viruses within seconds. The advantage of sanitizer is that you can use it without having to rinse again with water.

naturally, and about preventive medical treatment through seminars, online conferences and newly emerging clinical data. The best help I could get came from a friend in Pune (non-medical, from the armed forces) who sent me a steady supply of medicines and alerted me daily about new developments that I might miss. The other source of help was my brother (also from the armed forces). He provided me with a stack of N-95 masks and gloves and offered to buy me PPE clothing. The last, I declined because I was not working in a hospital environment where the risk of infection is much higher than it is for me. I do know that he supplied protective gear to a large number of medical staff who needed them. The role of these two army guys was far, far more important and genuine than the showy praise from the Armed Forces with helicopters showering flowers over hospitals, and serenading medical staff with music, thus expending Rs 68 crore. The banging of thalis and lighting lamps to ring in good health was just as empty a gesture.

I spoke to the district health officer at the beginning of the lockdown to find out if he had some guidelines for independently working practitioners like me. 'Madam…age…I advise you to shut the clinic and stay safe at home.' But I was one of the three doctors working in our town and one doctor became Covid positive and had to stay off duty for a long time. We two doctors catered to patients from many of the outlying villages and the town. The gentle warning from the DHO aside, no one interfered with my work; nor did I get any guidelines. There must be hundreds of doctors around the country who relied on their own resources to handle the pandemic in their areas. Such small, self-regulated efforts were an essential part of the rural struggle to cope with the crisis.

There has been enough evidence from several countries on the effective use of simple, safe oral medicines that can be given to patients quarantined at home. The front-runner among such drugs has been Ivermectin, a drug discovered in 1976 by Campbell and Omura and used widely in tropical countries in the treatment of certain parasites and worms. In 2015 they were awarded the Nobel Prize for the discovery of Ivermectin. Its early use has been found to be highly effective in curing 76 per cent of patients with Covid-19. It is antiviral and anti-inflammatory. Only those who present with more serious symptoms like recurring fever, cough, breathing difficulty or decreased oxygen saturation needed blood tests, CT scan and hospital referral.

Ivermectin is useful as prophylactic therapy for family members and those who have been in close proximity to infected cases, and for all frontline workers in society, like the police, traffic inspectors, autorickshaw and taxi drivers, shopkeepers, vendors—all those who have to go out on work. I first tried hydroxychloroquine for myself, as a preventive, along with Vitamin C, Zinc and Vitamin D3 and then switched to Ivermectin.

Based on these facts, I devised my treatment strategy. Those who presented at my clinic with symptoms and signs of respiratory infection were given routine treatment for three to five days. If they did not recover within three to five days, blood tests were done to rule out bacterial infections, typhoid, dengue and malaria. If the tests pointed towards a viral infection, the patient was given the choice to either get tested for Covid-19 or to undergo a week's treatment which I would closely supervise, by having the patient or the family member report to me on alternate days. All such patients were counselled at length about the illness, the need for distancing from family members and isolation, even within their homes.

Many of the patients I treated were hypertensive, diabetic or had other causes of chronic ill health. Since most of them had been in my care for years, it was easier for me to convince them about their role in containing the disease. Only those who presented with more severe symptoms like florid lung infections, breathing distress or extreme fatigue were referred to the district hospital.

Of the sixty-odd patients whom I treated thus, three required hospital admission and care for respiratory distress and declining oxygen levels. One among them was a diabetic with advanced renal disease and already on regular dialysis. The family were financially bereft and he expired within a week after developing the infection but his wife who got infected, recovered, in spite of being a poorly controlled diabetic. Another was found to have tuberculosis underlying the Covid infection. His condition improved after starting appropriate treatment for both but he is not yet fully recovered. The third, also a diabetic with heart disease, is lost to follow up.

*

The Covid-19 pandemic exposed clearly, the errors made by our government, the most fundamental being to rely entirely on Western wisdom in dealing with it and then rushing into an ill-timed lockdown, announced a mere four hours before enforcement. (South Africa gave four days' notice before locking down and Bangladesh gave a week.) Our government did not even consider the hundreds of million migrant workers who were stranded in cities and towns all over the country, with no jobs, shelter, transport home and food. It caused a humanitarian, social and economic debacle of huge proportions. The judiciary delayed hearing the many petitions that were filed against the government for causing this tragedy while those in power underplayed the ill effects of the monstrous goof-up. Everywhere across the country, ordinary citizens, NGOs, a few celebrities and corporates went out of their way to help to these distressed migrant workers.

These harsh truths were cleverly concealed under a blitzkrieg of self-congratulatory exaggerations of India's success in controlling the pandemic.

A year after it laid siege in most parts of the world, the virus appeared to be exiting. Effective vaccines were being made available, and India started its vaccination drive with much enthusiasm. So much so, we offered to help other countries with vaccines. For a brief period of six to eight weeks in January and February of 2021, there was a revival of activity and optimism. I had my first dose of vaccine and soon after went for lunch at my sister's. There was joy in wearing something nice after a year, meeting friends and family and yes, seeing people smile and laugh. It was all happening.

The possibility of a second wave due to new mutant strains was talked about as early as December 2020 and the likelihood of it happening in April-May 2021 in India was foretold by medical experts. It was also publicized in the news media. The government and the public failed to heed the warning. February and March 2021 saw the opening up of tourism, of restaurants, industries, the celebration of religious festivals, weddings and parties. India was literally beaming with pride at having come through the pandemic with fewer casualties than many of the Western countries. We congratulated ourselves on our genes, our immunity, our use of natural herbs.

The media was agog with excitement over election rallies, festival gatherings, religious pilgrimage to Hardwar by lakhs of Indians with no regard for the pandemic social precautions. Photographs of union ministers, a chief minister, sadhus and eager pilgrims taking a holy dip in the Ganga are fresh in my mind.

So right until early April 2021, as the Kumbh Mela progressed, saffron reigned. But within days, the same colour was mirrored in the cremation pyres—not merely in the vicinity of the Kumbh rituals but in all parts of the country. Thanks to a Kumbh returnee, a village near my home saw a swell of cases and many deaths. Apparently, this well-meaning devotee visited many homes to distribute prasadam and to regale them with his experience of the 'grandeur' of the Kumbh. This was soon followed by an annual, very popular village festival where everyone gathered. Within a week, tragedy struck and lives were lost. I had to shut my clinic yet again and see patients at home: many of them through an open window and others on the narrow front-porch. If I had to physically examine the patient (usually for lung signs and blood pressure and oxygen levels only at present) I wore a visor in addition to the mask.

*

Our battle with the Covid-19 virus has not been a very triumphant one. It is true that the 'Spanish Flu' which raged through the world for two years from early 1918 till the end of 1919 was more devastating. But surely, it is no comfort to find that hundred years on, we in India have such a wobbly and unequal health care structure that we have ceded so easily to its onslaught, resulting in the loss of lakhs of *preventable* deaths.

I stress on the word preventable. We started veering off the path of equitable health care from as early as the 1980s, we did not invest in improving the government-run public health system. Instead, we took the easy way out and privatized every aspect of health, we made health care a business enterprise. A business runs on profit; the more the better. You cannot escape the fact that a creaking government health system and a greedy private sector spell doom in times of real crises such as the one we are going through. When government hospitals began to fill up, the private sector was roped in. Finding that Covid-19 sufferers were the only 'captive' clients on offer, the private sector (facing the prospect of huge losses) admitted and overtreated many of those who were affected by the virus while more or less ignoring those who needed minimal but early and effective treatment. Intravenous antivirals were pumped in regardless of the necessity or proof of efficacy of most of these drugs. When patients deteriorated, steroids were used in large doses; the ICUs filled up with patients on oxygen and ventilator support. It is puzzling that well into the more devastating second wave, we had no universal guiding policy regarding treatment which can be made compulsory in all hospitals. The All India Institute of Medical Sciences (AIIMS) New Delhi and ICMR have regulated guidelines but they are not followed through effectively.

The lack of understanding of the difference between the first and second stages of the disease has led to sheer confusion, over-treatment, no-treatment, needless admissions and loss of manifold lives. Even in a small district like ours, there has been no attempt to link the various people in the health sector so knowledge and resources can be shared and used for collective betterment. If the treatment during the first stage is early and proper, only a small percentage (about 15 per cent) will reach the second stage of inflammation in the lungs and potential clotting dysfunction.

The objective is to detect cases as early as possible and initiate treatment. Of late, based on the experience of doctors worldwide, I use Ivermectin with a few other medications which are highly effective in bringing about a quick resolution of the disease. These are Doxycycline, Budesonide inhaler, Bromhexine, Fluvoxamine, Famotidine and antihistamines. I have stopped doing blood tests in all patients and do blood count, C-Reactive Protein (inflammatory marker), and blood sugar in all those who do not respond within a week. A raised CRP, spiking temperature in spite of treatment are indications for using steroids and a blood thinner in the appropriate dosage. I do not think a CT scan is essential for starting the second stage treatment especially in areas where facilities are few. If oxygen levels are okay, this can be done at home but if oxygen starts to dip at all, I prefer to send them to hospital for CT scan and constant monitoring, oxygen, etc.

While steroids are being touted as the only wonder drugs

for cure of Covid-19, it is imperative that they are not used as the first line of treatment as then they will do serious harm and no good. It is appalling to see chemist shops recommending steroid tablets and steroid injections to the gullible.

The questions that still remain unanswered are: Why have the simple measures used in combating the virus not been checked out more vigorously? Why do we dismiss simple drugs when their efficacy has been proved in large and widely reported clinical trials? Why does WHO repeatedly dismiss the use of Ivermectin, saying there isn't enough proof? Why are we drumming up the frenzy for vaccine as the only answer, knowing that it will take eight to ten months for Indians to be adequately protected by it? Till then do we carry on as we have done for eighteen months, for then, if a third wave happens, we will lose an unbelievable number of our people.

It is possible with the early and judicious administration of Ivermectin (along with Fluvoxamine as recently recommended) to avoid most of the hospital admissions, the use of expensive anti-virals of doubtful efficacy, CT scans, oxygen dependence, ICU care and even death. But the avoidance could be because hospitals need money. With their routine work having come to a near-standstill, they are probably desperate to revive hospital revenue. I don't know. Several months after the pandemic struck, the ICMR endorsed the use of Ivermectin along with other simple medicines but it failed to publicize it widely. These simple medications did not get enough coverage in the media as opposed to drugs like Remdesivir and Favipiravir both of which have hardly any value. Perhaps they were being cautious because there had been no extensive peer-reviewed clinical trials in the use of these medicines for Covid-19 infections. But any reasonably experienced general practitioner will tell you that we have used Ivermectin safely for years to treat *other* medical conditions. So the question of safety does not come in.

To add to it, there is the issue of vaccinations. Amidst

increasing fears about the duration of protection from the vaccines, it is now certain that we will be unable to vaccinate an adequate number of our population for at least eight to ten months, probably more. It is unlikely that the virus will be charitable enough to stop mutating further, causing another deadly surge at a time when at least a third of our population is nutritionally deficient.

If more virulent mutations do not occur, the coming year might be a hopeful one. But that is a big if. The early bungling, and the refusal to admit to it and address the tragedy caused has left millions in poor health due to undernutrition and malnutrition. Compounding the tragedy was a budget which did not show any increase in spending on public health infrastructure; and the new labour laws which will further curtail the rights of the labour force, while favouring the employers. The aftermath of the Covid years will shape the future course of our nation. One can only hope that we will have learnt important lessons from our failure.

32

A World View

Food, health, education and housing are the four essential needs of any society. It is little wonder then that every one of them has embraced the business model. We have high and low-end means of satisfying hunger and greed. There are centres of learning which snatch up kids as young as three, there is housing that is temporary or permanent of every size, shape and slickness; and there is health care.

We seek health in great earnest and little understanding, with the hope that the medical system can sort it all out. The health industry is a dynamic business offering fine-tuned expertise to the sick. It is a special domain of knowledge and skill for saving lives. But there is a problem.

The doctor who treats simple ailments without resorting to tests and referrals will soon be a curiosity. This, in spite of the fact that 90 per cent of our ailments are simple and easily curable. Where do you go when you are unwell? Who is to tell you whether yours is an easily curable illness or a serious one? How many general physicians does an area need, how many specialists and where? We have 542 medical colleges in the country. The government has plans to authorize 164 new colleges in the near future which will result in a total of 100,000 doctors graduating every year. There are 20,000 practitioners in the alternate systems. We need more doctors but it is clear that merely increasing the numbers does not work, as doctors tend to concentrate in urban areas.

Much of this has to do with policies which allowed a government-funded welfare system to be overtaken by the private sector. There has been no resistance to this change, because as a society, we are not particularly concerned with the idea of equitable health care that reaches all, we are merely concerned with our own health. We accept the unsatisfactory nature of governmental health care because we don't depend on them. We see a socialized welfare system as an outdated model. As long as we can purchase health with money power, we need not care about this public-private dichotomy. But it happens to be the lifeline for 75 to 80 per cent of our people who, after spending money on food, housing and the education of children, have precious little to spend on health.

Why should we (the fortunate 20 per cent) care?

Because: The private sector is focused on curing an illness that has already gripped the body. This is true in all parts of the country, both urban and rural. It does nothing to prevent illness, nor does it take responsibility for chronic, debilitating, serious diseases like tuberculosis or leprosy. It does not offer succour to the malnourished millions, the anaemic mothers and all those whose health is badly dented by the scourge of poverty. It is not their job. They are, almost always, profit-making ventures. Two thousand Indians die every day of tuberculosis and yet, this figure does not make us uncomfortable in the least.

The government must take a large share of the blame for ignoring the warning signals of a mismanaged health care system and encouraging its rapid privatization at the risk of social welfare. It is not impossible to reorganize and revive the system so it reaches all our people. The current government which does excellent publicity for itself is surely and steadily bringing in reforms which will suffocate equitable health care altogether. Interference at every level without clarity regarding the outcome of such changes, is dangerous. In recent years we have seen the revamping of the Medical Council of India, the ramping up of health insurance policy very similar to the disastrous policy of the US, encouraging private practice over socialized welfare and the attempt to permit doctors of Ayurveda to perform surgery.* A better idea will be to encourage alternate systems by setting up departments in every hospital where one can opt for alternate therapies. To make a khichdi out of assorted medical systems is to lose the treasure-house/s of ancient knowledge while adulterating surgical expertise at every level.

It is only now, when the Coronavirus pandemic brought the scare right into our homes that we have woken up to the reality that the infrastructure of our medical system is in tatters; we have understood why it is important to prevent an illness rather than wait until it needs a cure.

Our Public Health System is in tatters. It needs more attention than any specialized branch of medicine, because only an effective system which looks at the entire gamut of disease precursors like the unclean environment, polluted water, adulterated food and poisonous air can save the medical system. The pandemic has brought this into sharp focus.

Even so, there is no sense of urgency about setting right what is wrong. The government, they say, is well-intentioned. Everyone is well-intentioned but intent is not all. You cannot tighten a screw here, loosen a nut there, hammer in a few nails, coat it in Asian paint or whatever and resurrect a crumbling house.

---

*The craft of cutting and sewing can be learnt by any of us but craft is the least important part of being a surgeon. S/he works on living bodies, so what is crucial is the true understanding of what comes before and after the surgery. How does one decide when to cut, when not to cut? How does one prepare a patient for different types of surgeries? During surgery, how deep to go, how much pressure to apply on a squishy bit of bowel, an artery or nerve? What does the post-operative care consist of? How about the anaesthetist, is she also an Ayurvedic doctor? Lastly, will our very same politicians allow themselves and their dear ones to be operated thus? VIP volunteers, kindly step forward.

I have tried to give here, an idea of how medical systems work in other parts of the world. The National Health Service or NHS, first started in the UK, is the most equitable healthcare system in the world.* Canada, Australia and New Zealand have established a socialized system of medical welfare, based on the NHS. The economic status (or any status) of a person does not affect the quality of care. Doctors are salaried and therefore not under monetary pressure. The Scandinavian countries have similar systems in place.

In the last fifty years the US has raced past European nations to become the leader in medical advances, pharmaceuticals and biotechnology. Some of the best medical schools, hospitals, medical research centres and specialists are in the US. The country has had more Nobel laureates in the field of science than any other, even though several of them are the more recent immigrants. In spite of these merits, health care in the US is over-specialized, unequally distributed and less efficient than in other developed countries. It ranks forty-second among 191 nations in health indices (measured by life expectancy, infant and maternal mortality, chronic heart and lung disease, sexually transmitted disease, major accidents and obesity.) The US trails Chile (ranked thirty-fifth) and was snapping at the heels of Cuba (thirty-seventh) when I last checked, and is well behind Canada, Australia, New Zealand, UK, Japan, Germany, Switzerland, Netherlands, Norway and Sweden.

This is why: Health care in the US is largely private, and controlled by the insurance companies, called Health Maintenance Organizations or HMOs. They provide 'medical cover' according to the patient's ability to pay an annual premium. The HMOs monitor the cost of treatment and ensure that it stays well within the premium paid. Doctors report every case to the HMO who controls decisions like the

---

*See chapter 11 for a more detailed understanding.

length of hospital stay, the number of diagnostic tests that can be done and whether surgery can be undertaken if the need arises. In other words, they dictate terms to the doctors, thus shackling their decision-making capacity. Doctors are rewarded bonus payments when they do not incur wasteful expenditure, that is, when they do not treat patients who pay low premiums. The insurance companies hire an extensive administrative staff to devise ways of paying out less. One-third of every health-care dollar in the US is spent on insurance bureaucracy. It is little wonder that HMOs are as detested as tobacco firms.

The US is one of the few industrialized nations that does not guarantee health care to its people, although the amount of money spent on health is much more than in any other country. Prescription drugs are very expensive and for many citizens, neither the government nor the insurer will cover the cost of such drugs. Medical expenditure is a common reason for bankruptcy in the US. To quote Dr David Himmelstein of Harvard Medical School and the lead author of a study on health insurance: 'Unless you're Bill Gates, you're just one serious illness away from bankruptcy.' An exaggeration that is close to the truth. Indians residing in the US often get their various medical, surgical and dental problems fixed while holidaying in India. 'I would pay ten times this, in the US,' is what they tell you, talking about prices which make most of us *feel* ill. The irony of this situation is lost on everyone.

Forty-five million US citizens are unable to afford insurance. Their number is increasing in proportion to the increase in insurance premiums. They are mainly the Blacks, Hispanics, Asians and other minority immigrants who accept low-paying jobs which may not come with sickness benefits. This leads to their working even when sick, thus diminishing the quality of work. Sixty per cent of the medical practitioners in the US are in specialized medicine and 40 per cent deliver primary care.

There are Federal hospitals for the military personnel and the

Veterans Hospitals to look after them post retirement. All other citizens from low-income groups are treated at government-run hospitals which are ill-equipped and understaffed, with patients being cared for by junior doctors who are in search of better prospects.

The high level of dissatisfaction with the medical system has led to suspicion directed at the doctors. The belief—not altogether wrong—that doctors make a killing out of their ability to heal has resulted in rising medical litigations, even for flimsy reasons. Doctors have to take expensive insurance cover themselves to guard against litigation which is not unlikely in the course of a professional career.

The Affordable Health Care Act of 2010, also referred to as Obama Care, was designed to introduce a fairer form of insurance treatment that would include the poor and the uninsured while also setting up regulations that monitor the way insurance agencies work. Obama's successor, who did not believe that government has a responsibility towards the poor, dismantled the Act.

There are a few independent organizations in the US (one of the largest being run by the Kaiser Foundation) which offer a carefully planned health-care system designed to suit the patient, the medical practitioner and the insurance agency.

Germany has one of the best health-care systems in the world in terms of quality and cost. Two hundred and forty insurance agencies—which are called 'not-for-profit sickness funds'—work with groups of doctors to provide medical cover to 90 per cent of people at a cost that is half that in the US. The remaining 10 per cent take private insurance. The insurance providers are tightly regulated by the government towards socially desired ends. Drug manufacturers are also closely scrutinized. Any rise in the cost of a drug has to be justified with proper research and clinical proof of its superior value in comparison to existing drugs.

Doctors work privately, in groups, and are paid by the insurance agency with which they negotiate an annual budget and then work within that budget. Thus it self-regulates against any wasteful procedures and expense. The insurance premium paid by an individual is a fixed percentage of the income and is not related to the age of a patient, or the risk of disease. The government revenue covers children and the aged. On an average, the doctors in Germany earn a third less than those in the US.

China, Russia, Cuba and several other communist and socialist countries have fairer systems of health care than either the US or India. The state-run hospitals are free or subsidized, well maintained and properly equipped. The average citizen in these countries is healthier than the average Indian or American. A few years ago, a husband and wife couple (our close friends) were holidaying in Beijing when the wife fell seriously ill (with suspected brain haemorrhage). She was admitted to one of the leading hospitals for treatment. She stayed there for several weeks and returned to India only when it was safe to do so. They had no problem in getting the best doctors without any delay and although they paid for their treatment, they were very happy.

Several countries around the world have used more effective means of health-care delivery. Costa Rica is a middle-income country with the best health parameters in Latin America, and one of the best in the world. It has a publicly funded insurance policy which caters to all the citizens. The working population contributes 15 per cent of its salary for the scheme but even the unemployed can access it in a variety of ways. It provides total health care without any distinction between classes. The per capita expenditure on health is 562 dollars. Life expectancy is seventy-eight years and under-five mortality is 11 per 1000.

The success of the Costa Rican system is partly due to the large number of middle-level health workers who are cheaper than doctors and trained in providing effective health care. Because of long waiting lists, there are many who opt to get treated privately. So there is this alternative by which a citizen can get private consultation from a physician of his choice by paying a fee and still avail of insurance coverage for the investigations and most of the treatment.

Cubans had enjoyed a comprehensive health system since the 1960s. Its efficacy was undermined thirty years later when the Soviet Union and the Eastern Bloc, the biggest markets for Cuban products, disintegrated. The prolonged economic sanctions enforced by the US made it worse. Today their health system is in urgent need of a rehaul, with better availability of drugs, equipment and resources. But viewed from our own pitiful position, their health indicators are superior. The per capita expense of health is 229 dollars, life expectancy is seventy-six years and the under-five mortality, 9 per 1000.

Spain, with a life expectancy of seventy-nine years and under-five mortality just 6 per 1000, has done very well with its nationalized health service. Set up in 1986 by the socialist government, it offered universal coverage, free primary care, active prevention and promotional programmes. Eighty per cent of the people claim to be happy with the treatment in public hospitals. When the conservatives took over in 1996, there was a gradual dismantling of this service by decreasing expenditure, privatizing of laboratories, the use of high-tech diagnostics and an increase in private insurance companies. But there is also the healthful sign of strong public opposition to this conversion of a basic right into a merchandise.

Nearer home, Malaysia won world recognition from WHO and other international agencies for its health-care programmes. The government-controlled health service is financed by taxes and other public revenues which make it possible to provide extensive medical coverage in urban and rural areas. Health centres or the *Klinik desa* provide excellent primary care. The per capita expenditure on health is 345 dollars, life expectancy is seventy-five years and under-five mortality, 8 per 1000. However, their cash-strapped public system is considering privatization and ironically, along the failed American model. Senior staff, looking for more lucrative salaries, are being sucked into private hospitals, resulting in a lack of doctors and staff so essential for universal health care.

Sri Lanka offers the most relevant comparison for India. The per capita expenses on health in this island nation is 122 dollars, life expectancy seventy-two years and the under-five death rate, 19 per 1000. Malaria and malnutrition are being tackled in earnest. Sixty per cent of the outpatient and 95 per cent inpatient expenses are borne by the public sector. The government hospitals offer Ayurvedic and Allopathic care. There is focus on spreading awareness about public health and prevention of diseases: the abode of King Ravana, an underrated Shiva bhakta, has stolen a sprint over the holiest of holy lands which celebrates King Rama. Sri Lanka has recently been declared free of malaria, while India still carries a huge burden of this disease. This was possible because they have been able to eradicate the disease-carrying mosquitoes, with improved methods of public sanitation.* Even so, these benefits are yet to reach some remote areas in the country. The ethnic conflict of the last few decades and the increased spending on defence have made it more difficult. Privatization is encouraged but not at the cost of a good public system.

India is all set to imitate the failed insurance-based medical system of the US when there are better examples we could consider. The few government-based insurance schemes which operate in some states are poorly regulated and offer their services to a small number of people; the reimbursement of

---

*A Sri Lankan writer I met last year told me that she loves coming to India but the only thing she detests is the filth.

costs incurred by the hospitals in treating insured patients is delayed for months or years, resulting in diminishing quality of care; rural and small-town hospitals are not equipped with the administrative staff required to make insurance schemes truly beneficial; needless elective surgeries like Caesarean section, hysterectomy, cardiac and orthopaedic procedures are performed by hospitals to make easy money.

I am an Indian of modest means. I choose my doctors carefully, in order to get good treatment within my budget. If I had to pick between India and the US to be a patient in, I would choose India. Here the doctors are more easily accessible and unless you want to impress yourself with medical posh, you can still find good-quality treatment without spending too much. However, for certain types of super-specialized care, one has to seek the best among them and then there can be no compromise regarding the costs. This remains an unaffordable luxury for most of us.

If much of what I have said about the medical system sounds like a dirge, I take the blame for saying it. Only, I must remind the reader that the system is part of a whole: the country. We the citizens make it or break it. We are caught in the crosshairs of an unhealthy mix of private, governmental and insurance-based methods, with a touch of alternate medical therapies adding to the confusion. When implemented with prudence and fairness, each of these methods have proved their worth. India is a heavily populated country of 13.6 crore people. It must make room for socialized welfare as well as private, insurance-based medicine. After all, an efficient and equitable system translates into better health for the people, and comfortable earnings for the doctors.

Afterword

Self-portrait is exhibition of the self. So, it follows, that it should also be impeachment and defence. Your healer, your deliverer-from-suffering, your armed force, your pipe-cleaning angel and safai karmachari is but one trying to do what needs doing. You have just seen the sincerity and the deception, the valour and the cowardice beneath the white coat.

Acknowledgements

To Ravi Singh, for getting me to start the book, reminding me to keep at it (every few years) and ensuring the finish.

To Jerry Pinto, for reading and giving me his very valuable suggestions.

To Radhika Shenoy, for working on the final edit with skilled expertise.

ALSO IN SPEAKING TIGER

ONE FOOT ON THE GROUND

A Life Told Through the Body

Shanta Gokhale

In this unusual, extraordinary autobiography, Shanta Gokhale—writer, translator and one of India's most illuminating cultural commentators—traces the arc of her life over eight decades through the progress of her body, as it grows, matures and begins to wind down. Starting with her birth in 1939—in philosophic silence, till the doctor's slap on her bottom made her bawl—she recounts her childhood, youth and middle and old age in chapters built around the many elements and processes of the physical self: tonsils and adenoids, breasts and misaligned teeth; childbirth and fluctuating weight, cancer and bunions. And through these memories emerge others, less visible but just as defining: a carefree childhood growing up in a progressive Marathi household in Mumbai's Shivaji Park; the pleasures, in adolescence, of badminton, Kathak and hairdressing; the warmth of friends and an almost love in cold England; finding and losing a mate—twice—and bringing up her children as a single parent; the great thrill of her first translation from Marathi into English; nursing her mother, dying of cancer, as she would a baby; surviving cancer herself, and writing her second novel through the recovery.

Told with effortless humour and candour, *One Foot on the Ground* is the story of a life full of happiness, heartbreak, wonder and acceptance. It will rank among the finest personal histories written in India.

[illegible]

Nayana Goradia

In this unusual [illegible]

[illegible]

ALSO IN SPEAKING TIGER

THE BRASS NOTEBOOK

A Memoir

Devaki Jain

In this no-holds-barred memoir, renowned feminist economist and academician Devaki Jain recounts her own story and also that of an entire generation and a nation coming into its own. She begins with her childhood in south India, a life of comfort and ease with a father who served as dewan in the Princely States of Mysore and Gwalior. But there were restrictions too, that come with growing up in an orthodox Tamil Brahmin family, as well as the rarely spoken about dangers of predatory male relatives.

Ruskin College, Oxford, gave her her first taste of freedom in 1955, at the age of 22. Oxford brought her a degree in philosophy and economics—as well as hardship, as she washed dishes in a cafe to pay her fees. It was here, too, that she had her early encounters with the sensual life. With rare candour, she writes of her romantic liaisons in Oxford and Harvard, and falling in love with her 'unsuitable boy'—her husband, Lakshmi Jain, whom she married against her beloved father's wishes. Devaki's professional life saw her becoming deeply involved with the cause of 'poor' women—workers in the informal economy, for whom she strove to get a better deal.

In the international arena, she joined cause with the concerns of the colonized nations of the south, as they fought to make their voices heard against the rich and powerful nations of the former colonizers. Her work brought her into contact with world leaders and thinkers, amongst them, Vinoba Bhave, Nelson Mandela, Desmond Tutu, Henry Kissinger, Amartya Sen, Doris Lessing and Iris Murdoch, her tutor at St Anne's College, Oxford, who became a lifelong friend. In all these encounters and anecdotes, what shines through is Devaki Jain's honesty in telling it like it was—with a message for women across generations, that one can experience the good, the bad and the ugly, and remain standing to tell the story.